A MIDWIFE
THROUGH THE
DYING PROCESS

A MIDWIFE THROUGH THE DYING PROCESS

Stories of Healing and Hard Choices at the End of Life

Timothy E. Quill, M.D.

The Johns Hopkins University Press

Baltimore and London

© 1996 The Johns Hopkins University Press
All rights reserved. Published 1996
05 04 03 02 01 00 99 98 97   5 4 3 2

The Johns Hopkins University Press
2715 North Charles Street
Baltimore, Maryland 21218-4319
The Johns Hopkins Press Ltd., London

Library of Congress Cataloging-in-Publication Data
will be found at the end of this book.

A catalog record for this book is available
from the British Library.

ISBN 0-8018-5516-0

In Memory of

Arthur Schmale

Teacher, Mentor,

and Friend

Home is where one starts from. As we grow older

The world becomes stranger, the pattern more complicated

Of dead and living. . . .

. . . .

. . . In my end is my beginning.

T. S. Eliot,
from "East Coker," in *Four Quartets*

Contents

Preface and Acknowledgments

NINE SOULS form the center of this manuscript. Cynthia, Robb, Mrs. Martinez, Mr. Williams, Mrs. Johnson, John, Mr. Kline, Jane, and Jules are no longer with us in body, but their spirits will live on in these stories, and in the hearts and minds of their loved ones. I am indebted to each of them for teaching me about what it means to be human. Their families and friends also helped bring these stories to life by generously providing details that had been unknown to me and by providing feedback about early drafts.

After a brief introduction, each of the next nine chapters tells the story of the life and death of one of these remarkable individuals. They are a diverse group—women and men, black and white, young and old, rich and poor—each with a strong interest in maintaining a coherent voice in his or her own care. The hard choices they faced were determined both by their unique personal values and by very arbitrary but profound effects of their diseases. Dying became a time of personal healing for several; as their bodies deteriorated they became more whole as persons. Yet as the illness progressed, each also faced anguishing choices, initially between treatment of the disease and relief of suffering and later between continued living under undesirable circumstances and death.

The choices, themes, and meanings that affected me most strongly in each story are briefly commented on at the end of each chapter. These commentaries are intended to stimulate reflection and introspection rather than to resolve or thoroughly analyze. Those who wish more in-depth exploration will find relevant references at the end of each chapter. Chapter 10 synthesizes some of what has been learned in these stories into a series of recommendations and challenges, again supported by references for interested readers.

Penny Townsend-Quill, my sharpest critic, most intimate colleague, best friend, and wife, spent endless hours editing the stories and sharpening the commentaries. Without her love, support, hard work, and collaboration this book would not have been possible.

My practice partners helped care for these nine patients. They and many other physician, nurse, social work, and clergy colleagues have helped me explore, understand, and struggle through the many end-of-life dilemmas that our patients face every day. I especially want to thank Betty Rabinowitz for sharing her experience with Jules, described in chapter 9.

Maria Milella, my administrative assistant and colleague, spent countless hours refining the manuscript. Marc LaForce, my boss and partner in the Department of Medicine at the Genesee Hospital, gave me the opportunity to explore these difficult issues in depth, sometimes under adverse circumstances. Such academic freedom and support are rare in today's environment.

The University of Rochester School of Medicine and Dentistry has a rich tradition of emphasizing the central importance of the doctor-patient relationship in the training of all students and residents. George Engel and Alvin Ureles have been my role models with regard to integrating biological, psychological, and social dimensions of illness through the medium of the patient's story of illness, and Art Schmale taught me how to apply this approach to the care of the dying. I could not have had better training.

Although the University of Rochester School of Medicine and its Department of Medicine do not necessarily share my views about end-of-life decision making, they supported my recent sabbatical in the Netherlands, where this manuscript was completed. My sabbatical was also made possible by a generous grant from an anonymous donor who felt strongly that suffering patients deserve a much louder voice in what happens to them.

My parents, Joe and Millie Quill, taught me about the value of critical thinking, commitment, and caring. They gave my brothers and me the privilege of an excellent education and the freedom to follow our own path. My daughters, Carrie and Megan, have had the benefit and burden of being introduced to death and dying at an early age because of my activism and writings. They have always been quietly curious and supportive both during extensive periods of writing and during my close encounters with the law and the media.

Finally, I want to thank Wendy Harris and Joanne Allen, my editors at the Johns Hopkins University Press, for their belief in the project, guidance, and technical support.

I am blessed to be surrounded by a rich array of talented, caring, supportive colleagues, friends, and family.

A MIDWIFE
THROUGH THE
DYING PROCESS

Introduction

MEDICINE IS A healing profession. Physicians and other health care professionals devote their careers to helping people live longer and function better. The single-minded fight for life has yielded enormous successes, yet it has left practitioners without a clear vision of their responsibilities when their patients are dying. Death seems antithetical to modern medicine—no longer a natural and inevitable part of the life cycle, but a medical failure to be fought off, ignored, and minimized. The dark side of this desperate battle has patients spending their last days in the intensive care units of acute hospitals, tubes inserted into every body part, vainly trying to forestall death's inevitability. No one wants to die, but when we really have to, there must be a better way.

When medicine's purpose is defined solely in terms of curing and prolonging life, there is no clear direction when a patient is dying. Yet, healing has more to do with caring for the person who is ill than with simply extending biological life. The illnesses of real people include a complex mix of personal history, values, and concepts of self, spirit, and community. Medicine's purpose should include helping persons become more whole and alleviating their suffering, as well as treating their diseases. This broader conceptualization allows more meaningful possibilities for treating all patients, but particularly those who are dying. Whereas there may not be anything one can do to extend biological life, there is almost always a potential to enhance quality and meaning. Such is the role of a medical healer.

Most people would agree that when further efforts to prolong life are futile, doctors should help patients try to achieve a "good death."

Controlling pain and other forms of physical discomfort is the basic medical objective. We should have no reluctance about the use of high-dose opioid pain relievers; our dying patients should not be allowed to suffer if we have the ability to provide relief. Once physical symptoms are managed, many patients can then focus their energy on other important issues unique to the individual. For some, it is an opportunity to reaffirm connections with family and friends and to resolve interpersonal conflicts. For others, it may be a time of spiritual reflection, of exploring the meaning of this life or the possibility of an afterlife. Sometimes none of this healing is explicit, but may be expressed by putting one's tool collection in order or perhaps by settling one's finances and wills.

The way people die cannot be determined by a set formula or fixed assumptions. The patient should be encouraged to take the lead, with health care workers providing support and technical guidance. Within the limitations of patients' clinical circumstances, interventions should depend in large measure on their wishes and values. This caring approach is often given its fullest expression in formal hospice programs, in which a multidisciplinary team of nurses, social workers, home health aides, physical therapists, clergy, physicians, and volunteers share their expertise to address the needs of dying patients and their families. With the support of such teams, overseen by skilled primary care physicians, dying can be made at least tolerable, if not always ideal, about 95 percent of the time.

When patients achieve good control of symptoms and use their remaining time to come together with their families, complete unfinished business, and eventually accept their inevitable death, we as health care providers feel privileged to participate. Yet it is important not to oversimplify or romanticize the process. Dying can also be dominated by challenges that defy simple solutions. Approximately 5 percent of terminally ill persons eventually reach a point at which their condition becomes agonizing and overwhelming in spite of comprehensive efforts to palliate. These relatively few patients who find themselves dying a "bad death" also deserve our attention, compassion, and responsive-

ness. A patient's agony may come from a particularly intractable physical symptom, or it may reflect predominantly psychological, social,
spiritual, or existential threats unique to that person. Sometimes a single aspect of suffering dominates; at other times it is an aggregate of several dimensions that collectively become intolerable. Although the
medical profession should always use its expertise to look for opportunities to be helpful, some kinds of severe suffering may not be re-
lievable by medical or psychosocial interventions.

The best way to get beneath the surface of the personal and ethical challenges of dying is through real-life patient narratives. Nine stories selected from my relationships with patients and colleagues form
the core of this book. Each story illustrates a critical aspect of the myriad dilemmas faced regularly by patients, families, and health care
providers. Rather than one moment in time, each story involves a series of difficult decisions, one following on the heels of another. Their
sequence and evolution provide a context for understanding the meaning and importance of subsequent decisions. Each of these patients
faced moments of truth in which the edges of the law and ethics were
tested. The meaning and the potential for resolution of each dilemma
can be appreciated only by knowing the patient's personal background
and the history of the relationship between the patient and his or her doctor. Isolating these decisions from their context undermines their full
understanding. Medical decisions are easy to second-guess from the comfort of the ivory tower. Grappling with them from inside a doctor-
patient relationship committed to partnership and nonabandonment
is a much more vital and important challenge.

Six of the nine patients whose stories are told here eventually
reached a point at which they preferred dying to continued living under
the conditions they were forced to endure. They were not suicidal as we
ordinarily understand this term. The image of self-destructiveness con-
noted by the word *suicide* does not capture the tragic circumstances of
these patients, who had heroically used modern medicine to live longer,
only to find themselves in a nightmare from which there was no escape. Death eventually became the only avenue for preserving what lit-

tle remained of their personal integrity. The notion that all requests to physicians for assisted death stem from undertreated pain, unrecognized depression, or some kind of character flaw is an illusion. The wish to die demands exploration. It may be a clue to a potentially remediable problem, but it may also be rational and consistent with the patient's values and clinical circumstances. When dying becomes dominated by disintegration and humiliation, we in medicine must learn to respond more creatively and with more immediacy than we currently do. The patient's personhood lies in the balance. Such dying should be nothing short of a medical emergency.

Unfortunately, current medical ethics and the law often make it dangerous to respond openly to patients in such dire circumstances. The safest thing for doctors to do is to minimize and even ignore their desperate requests, thereby abandoning them to act on their own or to continue suffering. Patients fear that their doctors will not help them if they reach a point in their illness that tests the boundaries of medical ethics and the law. Many have witnessed harsh deaths of friends or family members in which physicians were afraid to act. Most know from personal experience that dying in the real world is almost never neat nor without repeated challenges. Without the explicit commitment of a physician to see the process through wherever it goes, the patient's energy may be depleted by focusing on his or her fear of future suffering rather than on more meaningful spiritual, existential, or social processes.

I have made every attempt to remain true to the complex realities faced by these patients and their physicians. These stories are limited primarily by my perceptions and recollections, supplemented by medical notes, recorded interviews, and written materials provided by the patients' families. Many family members reviewed early drafts to ensure their accuracy. In some of the stories minor details and names have been changed to respect the requests of those who wish to maintain anonymity. Several patients gave their consent before they died for their stories to be used. In the cases of the other patients, permission was granted by the families, who believed their loved ones would want their story to be told. Each narrative is followed by a brief commentary on the central themes that emerged. These discussions are not intended to be exhaustive. My goal is to stimulate the reader to reflect on the dilemmas that were confronted rather than to resolve them. References are provided at the end of each chapter for those who want to explore a particular issue in more depth. In the final chapter, I outline eleven challenges that patients, families, physicians, ethicists, lawyers, and policy makers must address in providing a comprehensive system of care for the dying.

Commitments to partnership and nonabandonment are relatively easy to articulate in the abstract. Fulfilling them in the real, often messy drama of dying can be as daunting as it is rewarding. When death was imminent, and suffering severe, solutions were found that balanced the needs and values of patient, family, and doctor in the context of current ethical and legal constraints. Some of the endings had all of the elements of a "good death," whereas others were painfully inadequate; they were simply the best we could do under the circumstances. These patients and their families had no choice but to endure the terminal phase of their illnesses. Our burden and our privilege as health care providers is to go through it with them. For me, this commitment reaffirms why I became a physician. Although it is often characterized by uncertainty and imperfect solutions, helping people die well is as important as helping them in the fight for life and recovery.

Chapter 1

"A Midwife through the Dying Process"

CYNTHIA APPEARED VIBRANT, alive, and engaging. It was hard to believe that at age thirty-seven she was already desperately ill. Exceptional in so many ways, she had done all the right things to take proper care of herself. She was a vegetarian who kept herself physically fit. She was enrolled in a doctoral program in psychology, studying whether beliefs about an afterlife affect how people live in the present. Her spiritual practice of Zen Buddhism included regular meditation and self-reflection. She had recently fallen in love with someone who shared her values and interests, and she was making deep connections with her colleagues, students, and friends. How could someone this healthy have contracted such a severe illness?

Cynthia's life had not always been filled with joy and clear purpose. She had been a rebellious adolescent; to her parents' chagrin, she had temporarily dropped out of high school. She felt stifled by educators who tried to control rather than bring out her creativity and intelligence. Cynthia needed to determine her own path. If she made mistakes, at least they would be her own. Cynthia's parents were terrified by her newfound autonomy, but they soon learned that efforts to extinguish her drive for independence only made it stronger. Her father, himself a person of no small will, had a particularly hard time accepting her nontraditional choices. Yet Cynthia demonstrated at every turn that her emerging self would not be thwarted.

Cynthia eventually returned to high school and then went on to college. She found that her gifts as a teacher included a unique ability to reach out to learners who had been labeled "difficult." Cynthia discovered the importance of allowing students at all stages of development to define part of the educational agenda and build upon rather than dominate their inner curiosity. While she continued to struggle with those in authority, she could always find satisfaction in fostering the inner strengths of students with all sorts of disabilities and limitations. Although the teaching programs she was involved in were always nontraditional, she received awards and citations for excellence at every turn.

Cynthia was raised in a Quaker household. To no one's surprise, her spiritual beliefs assumed dimensions far from her family's tradition. She eventually gravitated to the Zen Center in Rochester, New York, where she lived for several years. In Zen Buddhism Cynthia found the freedom and discipline to continue her inward journey. For the first time, she seriously considered the meaning of death and discovered more of what was important in life. Her mind had always been razor sharp, but her capacity for human connection and inner peace was furthered by her Buddhist practice. Her intellectual intensity began to find some spiritual balance as new dimensions of her being were explored.

Her journey had its ups and downs. There were periods when she felt lost and alone, wondering where she was going and with whom. A marriage came and went. Several teaching jobs that seemed fulfilling at first eventually fractured and fizzled. When the direction she wanted to take gradually became more defined, she enrolled in a doctoral program in psychology at the University of Rochester. In this setting, her interests in educational methods, spirituality, and empowerment could be integrated. The seemingly disparate parts of her life were finally coming together. Her professors, who shared her disdain for traditional educational methods, were engaged in the scientific study of the relative educational efficacy of enhancing versus controlling a learner's autonomy. Cynthia's initial research demonstrated that persons who had a more fully conceptualized sense of life after death had increased vitality and self-actualization in this life. (The irony and tragedy of her study topic were not lost on anyone as her illness unfolded.) Cynthia also fell in love with a fellow graduate student named Tim, who shared her values, intellect, and intense commitment to quality, as well as her disdain for authority. Life was full, and the future seemed limitless.

Cynthia was finishing her first-year courses and trying to interpret the data collected from her research project, when she became fatigued and developed an upset stomach. Initially attributing these symptoms to overwork, she resolved to take better care of herself, confident that the symptoms would disappear with appropriate rest. When they did not, she made an appointment with a doctor at the University Health Service. She was seen promptly, but she found the visit unsatisfying, feeling that the doctor had not taken her symptoms seriously enough. Her problem was attributed to a combination of heartburn and stress; antacids and rest would do the trick. Although Cynthia was irritated by the visit, she knew her response to authority well enough not to dismiss the doctor's recommendations out of hand. She dutifully took the antacids and followed the doctor's advice to get more rest with the expectation that she would soon recover.

Over the next ten days, however, her symptoms worsened. She began to lose weight, and swallowing became an ordeal. Cynthia saw another physician, who found an abnormal firmness in the top of her abdomen. Although he wasn't sure what it was, he immediately recommended blood tests and x-rays. When Cynthia asked about the possibilities, the doctor initially mentioned hepatitis or peptic ulcer disease. When she asked about the worst-case scenario, he tried to defer the discussion until after the tests had been obtained. Unable to contain her inquiry, Cynthia pushed harder for an answer, suggesting that her imagination would run wild if she didn't know the range of possibilities. The doctor reluctantly opened the door to the possibility of lymphoma, a cancer of lymph cells that can affect the stomach. He reassured her that in the unlikely event that it was lymphoma, it was a highly treatable, usually curable, cancer.

The x-ray of her stomach showed a large mass enveloping most of her stomach. In the discussion of the results peptic ulcer disease and hepatitis were ruled out as possibilities; lymphoma was the odds-on favorite. The doctor emphasized that while obviously no one wants to get cancer, lymphoma was a "good one" because of its responsiveness to treatment. Cynthia once again wondered what else it could be. The doctor allowed that gastric cancer was a remote possibility, but he said that it was almost unheard of in persons as young as Cynthia who did not have other genetic or environmental risks. When she asked what it would mean if she had gastric cancer, the doctor responded that, unlike lymphoma, "gastric cancer is a bad one."

Arrangements were made for a gastroenterologist to pass a tube into her stomach to do a biopsy. Cynthia's world was shaken, but she remained confident that she could cope with whatever came. Her worst-case scenario was that she would need surgery and perhaps chemotherapy. She could use the summer to recover and start school again in the fall. The first inkling that things didn't look good came after the stomach biopsy: the doctors, who had been so friendly before the procedure, were now distancing themselves, hands behind their backs, remote and unresponsive. Perhaps she was being too sensitive. Maybe her perceptions had been altered by the anesthesia. She went home with Tim for the agonizing three-day wait until the biopsy would be ready.

She was restless and unable to sleep. Her future, once so bright and clear, was now filled with uncertainty and doubt. Her imagination ran out of control; she dreamt of death and mutilation. What was the worst that could happen? How bad could it be? On the day before her appointment she could stand the uncertainty no longer. She telephoned her doctor. The doctor initially played for time, saying that the final report would not be out until the next day. Besides, it was not a good idea to discuss these matters over the telephone. His tone was worrisome, and Cynthia's mind went into overdrive.

"If the final report is not out, there must be a preliminary report?" she queried.

"Yes." The doctor was silent, hoping the conversation could be postponed.

"I really need to know because this waiting is driving me crazy," Cynthia pressed on.

"Are you sure you want to hear this over the telephone?" *I really don't want to do this right now,* he thought.

"Yes, I'm sure."

9

"Well, it is looking less and less like lymphoma," he hedged.

"Does that mean that its looking more and more like gastric cancer?"

"I'm afraid that it is."

Oh! My God! "Well, thank you for telling me."

Cynthia hung up. She felt more alone and terrified than she had ever felt before. She was in a free fall, a black hole, and the boundaries of just how "bad" it could be were nowhere to be found. In circumstances such as these the brain often mercifully shuts down and numbness and mild confusion dull the pain. She was by herself at first, which magnified her sense of aloneness in a world that had no landmarks. Tim arrived shortly thereafter. They hugged, cried, and searched desperately for the edges of her disintegrating world. Surgery, radiation, chemotherapy—which approach would the doctors recommend? None of the choices sounded appealing, but together the two of them would figure out how to cope and get on with their life.

Cynthia's appointment the next day was devastating. Her gastric cancer was very aggressive, involving her entire stomach and likely to have spread elsewhere. It was a *linitis plastica* cancer, and its characteristic *signet cells* carried a very poor prognosis. Her doctors had carefully researched the treatment options in the medical literature and had discussed her case with various specialists in medical and radiation oncology. Conventional treatment regimens were ineffective. She could try experimental therapy, but it would most likely only contribute to more suffering and not to prolonging her life. The course they were recommending was palliative care. They promised to do their best to keep her comfortable for the time that she had remaining and to provide pain medicine if necessary.

Cynthia couldn't believe that they were talking about her. "The fact that they would use the word terminal had not crossed my mind." She found no hope in their initial recommendation. Cynthia needed to find a way to fight her illness even if the odds were poor and the strategies radical. "There is a world of difference between no hope and a ray of hope! It's black and white, night and day." Though she accepted her diagnosis and just how serious it was, she could not accept the certainty of her prognosis. To accept palliative care at that point, without a medical fight, would have been toxic to her as a person. "They don't know who will live and who will die! They don't know! They don't know!" she raged. Although she knew that the odds of experimental therapy were very slim, she felt that even a tiny chance of success was better than a certain death sentence.

Cynthia saw herself, correctly, as an exceptional person. She reasoned that since gastric cancer was such a rare condition in someone her age, some of the reported statistics might not apply in her specific case. She had the statistical background to understand the odds, but she also knew that for each individual it is all or none. It works or it doesn't; life or death. She went directly to the medical literature and also researched alternative healing methods. Although much of what she found was not hopeful, she did find case reports of individuals who had beaten the odds in spite of a supposedly hopeless prognosis. In the midst of chaos and desperation, her hope and energy were rekindled by these reports. She began to visualize herself getting better, and she tried to find an approach that made sense.

Over the next ten days, which seemed like a lifetime, Cynthia talked to many doctors and alternative healers. She explored as many avenues as possible, but she was also wary of charlatans who might prey on her desperate situation. She felt tremendous pressure to make a decision, fueled by the belief that with each moment that she waited, the cancer could spread to a critical part of her body unreachable by treatment. In her darker moments her imagination would shift from healing to disintegration and decay. The uncertainty was at times overwhelming, but she persevered until her course began to become clear.

She eventually met a surgeon who was willing to work with her as a partner and to explore experimental treatment. She also became my patient at this time. Since her medical options were severely restricted, the most important things I could do initially were to listen to her story and help her analyze her clinical dilemma in all of its complexity. I also gave her some breathing room by assuring her that taking one to two weeks to make a sound decision was not going to alter her small chances of success.

We agreed to work together no matter what course she chose or what the outcome. As far as possible, I would keep her in the driver's seat of her medical treatment. Since conventional medical therapy had been proven ineffective in gastric cancer, experimental therapy was her only option for aggressive medical treatment. Yet, the odds of its prolonging her life, much less curing her disease, were remote. The experimental protocols being offered—radical surgical removal of the stomach and surrounding tissues, followed by aggressive chemotherapy—were toxic. Viewed optimistically, such therapy had one chance in one hundred of controlling the disease for anywhere from a few months to a few years. The odds of a cure would be much smaller. Conversely, the probability was 99 percent that the treatment would not work and her last weeks and months would likely be dominated by the side effects of futile medical intervention. This was Cynthia's reality.

How should I talk truthfully to Cynthia about such poor odds without depriving her of hope? She needed to understand the facts about aggressive treatment, as well as what she might be losing by forgoing a comfort-oriented approach from the outset. With comfort care, all medical interventions would be geared to relieving symptoms, improving the quality of life, and keeping her in control. It wouldn't preclude the possibility of a spontaneous remission, but it would encourage a broader search for hope and meaning beyond the small potential of traditional medical interventions to cure or prolong life. Although comfort-oriented care may have made the most sense from a purely statistical point of view, to Cynthia it initially made no sense to give up without a medical fight. If she had to die, she wanted to be able to take the time to prepare—a process for which comfort care is much better suited. But she could not prepare herself to die without at least trying to win this improbable medical battle. Otherwise the possibility that it might have worked would haunt her.

Once I was assured that Cynthia understood her choices and their potential consequences, I felt better about embarking on the experimental course. The scientific part of me knew that it was a long shot that might add to the suffering of a person who would die anyway of a terrible disease. Yet, there was also a very remote chance that it could work, and this clinical trial had become very important to Cynthia. She had no good choices. Having spent precious time and energy coming to grips with that unfortunate fact, she had chosen experimental treatment. It was now time for us to move forward, if not with enthusiasm, then at least with a clear sense of common mission.

Our preparatory work, however, was not yet complete. Cynthia wanted assurance that she could stop treatment in the future if it was no longer meeting her needs. The experimental protocol she was considering involved surgery followed, after a recovery period of several weeks, by intensive chemotherapy. Although she had agreed to the protocol, she was much more certain about the need for surgery than she was about the need for chemotherapy. She wanted to take time in the recovery period to better understand the drugs, including their potential side effects. She also wanted to try some nontraditional nutritional therapies, and she hoped this would not disqualify her from the experimental protocol.

From a medical, ethical, legal, and personal point of view, this was a relatively simple question. Patients have the right to refuse therapy if and when their goals or circumstances change. This is possible even when it is the case that they would live with certainty with therapy and die without it. These decisions should not be made lightly, but once informed consent is assured, physicians are obligated to support them. I reassured Cynthia that I would honor her decision to stop therapy if it no longer served her goals.

Many of those with superficial knowledge of Cynthia's thought processes viewed her choice of experimental therapy as part of her "denial of death." Given the magnitude of what she was trying to comprehend, there is probably a grain of truth to this speculation. Yet, Cynthia faced severe illness more squarely than most patients whom I have encountered. She talked openly about her worst fears and greatest hopes. Because of her Buddhist beliefs, Cynthia saw in death a natural and inevitable form of rebirth. The process of dying, on the other hand, filled her with trepidation. Being fully cognizant and able to connect both intellectually and emotionally with those around her were central to her concept of personhood. If these were lost, then her life would have no purpose. She also feared being a burden on others for a prolonged period and dying in severe pain. The quality of her life was more important to her than its quantity. She wanted to live only as long as she could find meaning and dignity and then be allowed to die peacefully.

Therefore, Cynthia also wanted reassurance that I would be willing to ease death if she found her condition too degrading, humiliating, or painful. In Zen Buddhism, how one dies has considerable bearing on how one is reborn in the next life. Being at peace is the best one can hope for, and dying in agony puts one at risk. I reassured Cynthia that modern palliative measures can relieve the vast majority of cancer pain. Large doses of opioid pain relievers could be provided if necessary, even in doses that might indirectly contribute to her death. Because of my past work as a hospice medical director, I have great confidence that I can address my patients' pain problems at the end of life. I promised Cynthia that I would do so without fear or restraint.

Reassuring her that I would help her find an escape if her dying became degrading or humiliating in domains other than pain was much more challenging. Some methods of easing death, such as stopping life-sustaining therapy or administering high-dose opioids for pain, are openly accepted in our society. Approaches in which death is more explicitly assisted, such as providing a dying patient with barbiturates that he or she can take if the suffering becomes overwhelming, are prohibited. Like many patients who fear a bad death, Cynthia was relatively unconcerned about the specific methods, provided they were effective. She simply wanted the assurance that I would work with her to find an acceptable way to die if she ended up in an intolerable condition toward the end. I made this commitment to Cynthia, as I do to all my dying patients. Usually, standard palliative care and hospice methods are effective when they are used in an individualized, creative fashion. Yet some patients, like Cynthia, need even more explicit reassurance that their suffering will not be ignored.

In an interview three weeks after her diagnosis Cynthia talked about a

> feeling that I got [talking to her surgeon and to me] that no matter what happened, if I did recover or if I didn't, that you wouldn't abandon me—that I was . . . more than just another case of gastric cancer coming through. . . . And to have somebody who was willing to stay there with me through all the possibilities, both the possibility of recovery (and that's where the hope comes in) and the possibility of not recovering, which means that you have to deal with that possibility. I mean, thinking that you have failed, and get beyond that and deal with that however you need to, and still be willing to stay with me. That's different from saying, "We can provide palliative care." I don't know how to explain that. I got the feeling that they would prescribe pain medicine for me but not that anyone would be willing to still have a relationship with me—a doctor-patient relationship with me—and midwife me through the dying process if that's what it came to.

This promise—to "midwife" patients through the dying process— is what most dying patients and their families want from their health care providers. It is at the core of hospice and other forms of palliative care. It implies allowing the full expression of the patient as a person in the face of very adverse life circumstances. Uncertainty about how the future will unfold makes severe, potentially terminal illness exquisitely frightening. If the course and its time frame could be known in advance, one could more easily prepare. But for Cynthia and countless others faced with a poor prognosis, the future poses unpredictable medical as well as spiritual, social, and psychological challenges. Therefore, the importance of going through it with a committed, experienced medical partner cannot be overstated.

Armed with these assurances, Cynthia felt confident enough to begin experimental therapy. This temporarily ended her free fall. The landmarks of her immediate future were defined. Although she could not anticipate all of the turns her life might now take, she felt she had collaboration with and support from her doctors. In spite of overwhelming uncertainty and fear at times, she also found her life assumed an intensity as never before. She related to people more directly than ever. Many friendships deepened and became more intimate in the face of her adversity. She no longer took any aspect of her life for granted, and she resented those people who still had the luxury to do so. Although this was not, of course, a path she would have chosen, she found some positives to compensate in a small way for her devastating losses.

Each member of Cynthia's immediate family came to grips with her illness in his or her own way. Her father dropped his own academic endeavors and went to the medical literature to try to understand the disease that had invaded his beloved daughter's life. When he didn't like the answers he found, he sought the opinion of a wide range of experts. He would leave no stone unturned. He believed that through hard work, diligence, and intellectual rigor a better approach would be found. Cynthia's mother was more in touch with the enormity of the loss and the need to stay supportive and strong for both her daughter and her husband. Tim tried to understand and maintain an openness to the reality that Cynthia faced. He joined with her in each step of the process, attending medical appointments and openly exploring options. Cynthia and Tim talked about anything and everything—avenues of hope as well as feelings of hopelessness—without forcing premature closure. Their love strengthened, and their commitment to see the process through together was reaffirmed.

Cynthia knew that there was a small chance that surgery or her disease might render her mentally incapacitated. If that happened, she wished to die as peacefully and quickly as possible. Because of her Buddhist beliefs, she felt that life without consciousness and the potential to connect with others was not worth living. Under such circumstances she would rather free her spirit to move on to the next life. She therefore completed a living will and named a health care proxy to represent her in medical decisions if she could not represent herself.[1] Tim would be her proxy, for Cynthia felt that he would have the strength to let her go if she lost her mental abilities in the future. These discussions about advance directives were emotionally laden for both Cynthia and Tim because they represented an open acknowledgment of her extreme frailty. Yet, they actually made Cynthia feel more secure as she faced treatments with very high risks and a disease known for its lethality.

The surgery was radical, and our unstated hopes that the disease might miraculously be localized were dashed. Her stomach was removed, and her esophagus was reattached to her small intestine. Visibly diseased lymph nodes in her abdomen were also removed, and we all knew that other tissues would inevitably be involved at a microscopic level. Tubes were placed in a central vein so that she could be given fluids and nutrition while her alimentary tract was recovering. Additional tubes were left in her small intestine for drainage and potential feeding and in her abdomen to allow the delivery of chemotherapy directly to her remaining intestines. Her body, which she had worked so hard to keep healthy, had been invaded, and the desperate fight was on.

In recovery Cynthia remained optimistic. She wanted to know the exact findings and their implications. Although most of the news was bad, the lack of visible liver involvement seemed to be a small bright spot. She wanted to get home, where she felt she could recover more quickly, and begin to explore nutritional therapy. We hoped to delay chemotherapy for four to six weeks so that she could prepare herself mentally as well as physically. She left the hospital with her hope undiminished but with a feeling of extreme vulnerability. The surgery had

---

1. The living will and the health care proxy are two forms of advance directives whereby one can define the medical care one would want if one lost the mental capacity to speak for oneself in the future. In a living will, one's own philosophy is set out, including the circumstances under which it would apply. Since not all possibilities can be anticipated, many also choose a health care proxy, a person to represent their wishes in health care decisions if they cannot speak for themselves. Sample forms and instructions about these advance directives are included in the Appendix.

been more invasive than she had anticipated. The true burdens and risks of the course she had chosen were beginning to sink in.

Cynthia's time at home was relatively short. Within two weeks her intestines had become obstructed from the relentless progression of her disease and she was back in the hospital needing emergency surgery. The cancer had spread throughout her abdomen. In spite of her weakened condition and her lack of emotional preparation, chemotherapy could not be further postponed if it was to have even a small chance of working. Her ray of hope was fading. Chemotherapy would be tried because of the slim chance that she might respond dramatically, but the likelihood that it would not help began to circle ever closer.

Chemotherapy was harsh. She had all the common side effects: nausea, vomiting, fever, low blood counts, weakness, and fatigue. Just as she began to regain her strength, it was time for another treatment. Her quality of life was rapidly deteriorating. We decided to repeat a CT scan of her abdomen after only two cycles of treatment. The members of the health care team were by now very connected with Cynthia, and we all eagerly anticipated the results—hoping for the best but expecting the worst. Unfortunately, we found what we expected. Her disease continued its rapid progression.

Before talking with Cynthia and Tim, I met with the oncologists to confirm my belief that further chemotherapy was futile. We explored other experimental avenues, especially those that might be relatively free of side effects. I wanted to be sure that I was aware of all the remaining medical options. The oncologists agreed that further medical treatment had no real chance of succeeding and would only diminish the quality of Cynthia's life. We knew that referral centers like the Memorial Sloan Kettering Cancer Center in New York City would probably offer further experimental therapy if she wished but that there was virtually no chance that it would help. Since our oncologists tend to be aggressive, and their advice was consistent with my own knowledge, I felt prepared to talk to Cynthia and Tim about the medical facts. Putting Cynthia through further treatment that induced rather than relieved suffering now made no sense at all. It was time to switch to a comfort-oriented approach and to allow her to direct her limited time and energy toward more humane and productive ends.

Cynthia had perceived past recommendations about palliative care as devoid of hope, so I approached the discussion carefully. That her condition was worsening and chemotherapy was not working came as no surprise to Cynthia or Tim. There was a sad finality to hearing it, but they had both been expecting the worst. I approached the conversation about referral to a hospice program slowly, listening to as well as watching their responses. I acknowledged that the last month had been extraordinarily difficult and that the treatments we all had hoped would help had only aggravated her suffering. I shared my belief that further aggressive medical treatment would be futile and recommended that we shift our energies exclusively to maintaining her comfort and dignity. The best approach would be a hospice program, in which the resources of a multidisciplinary team could be used to enhance her quality of life and help her stay at home if at all possible.

Cynthia and Tim were disappointed, but they were relieved that she didn't have to undergo further aggressive treatment. The prospect of going home appealed most to them. During Cynthia's stay in the hospital Tim had found a beautiful place in the country. A stream and small waterfall in the backyard provided an atmosphere of peace and serenity, which Cynthia craved. Cynthia was enrolled in a hospice program. Since she could not eat or drink, she elected to continue her intravenous feeding. Nutrition was very important to Cynthia, so the fluids used were full of nutrients, in spite of research data suggesting that hyperalimentation is not of medical value to cancer patients. She was also receiving a continuous intravenous infusion of morphine, which controlled her pain. She was not ready to die, but wanted to live only as long as her life remained meaningful to her. She had a lot of work to do to prepare for death, and she hoped she would have enough time to complete this process.

She called her parents to inform them of the latest developments. They left the following morning to come to Rochester. Having been spared some of the more agonizing moments of Cynthia's hospitalizations, they were not fully prepared to face this transition. Yet the degree of suffering she endured in her medical fight was not lost on them. They too courageously accepted the transition to hospice, thus acknowledging the tragedy that their daughter was dying. Cynthia's mother and father remained in Rochester, staying with relatives, so that they could be with her for the final phase of her illness.

Cynthia's hospice time was a rich experience for all those who were privileged to participate. She was initially able to take short walks along the backyard stream. The sights, sounds, and smells of her new rural home were so far removed from the stark, bland hospital room that for brief periods she could escape the reality fate had dealt her. Both her spiritual beliefs and the philosophy of the home hospice program encouraged her to focus on the present, taking the challenges as they came, one day at a time. She took this guidance to heart, gradually becoming the guide rather than the follower.

Cynthia had a directness and an articulateness that allowed her to transcend her bodily limitations and experience other people in an intensely human and open way. She began the process, simultaneously wonderful and agonizing, of preparing for death. When she first went home, her energy level was relatively high and she met with her closest friends and family to say what needed to be said. She gave her favorite possessions to special people in her life so that they would have something to remember her by. Cynthia and Tim married in a small ceremony—Cynthia in bed and Tim by her side, where he would remain for her last weeks. Members of the Buddhist community came to their house several times each week for a group meditation. As she grew weaker, Cynthia repeatedly said that she found group presence in shared meditation without the burden of words to be the most energizing engagement for her. Non-Buddhists friends were invited to participate, and there was a rare sense of community and spirituality in which we all could partake. Her parents, who visited daily, learned to connect with her without trying to take over. The hospice nurses all commented that the opportunity to work with patients like Cynthia was what had drawn them to this type of work in the first place.

I too visited regularly and was made a part of the spiritual journey that Cynthia was creating out of chaos. It was wonderful to witness how her spirit soared as her body deteriorated and how those around her were growing in the process. But my visits also had a medical aspect—a challenging, often primitive counterpart to the processes of personal growth and connection. Cynthia's clinical condition was rapidly deteriorating; she had increasing pain, nausea, and vomiting, and an open wound filled with cancer was growing on her abdomen. During each visit we would address these symptoms in the hope that they could be controlled sufficiently to allow the extraordinary process of her saying good-bye to continue. I regularly increased the level of her morphine infusion, which successfully suppressed her pain most of the time. We tried a variety of antinausea treatments, which temporarily, at least, subdued her vomiting if not the nausea. After consulting with several experienced hospice nurses, we developed a mixture of antibiotic powder and antacids that countered the smell emanating from her open wound. One day at a time, I reminded myself.

I tried to keep myself, as well as Cynthia and her family, focused on the present and not on the future.

"How long do I have?" One of the dreaded questions asked of doctors, both by patients and by their families (as we move just out of hearing range).

"I don't know."

"But what do you think?"

I try to be honest, while always leaving room for the unexpected. "Probably not too long—a few weeks, maybe a month or two, though there are exceptions in either direction."

"How bad do you think it will get?"

"It is hard to know, but we will work together to find solutions, no matter what happens."

My commitment was reaffirmed, but I too wondered what Cynthia's future would bring, and I wondered what might be required of me. So far it had been an uplifting, spiritually fulfilling process. My hope was that she could die with peace and acceptance and that only standard hospice measures would be required. Dying can be a meaningful clo-sure to a family's coming together and to a person's completing his or her life trajectory, but on occasion the challenges posed by the dying process can threaten the very fabric of what it means to be a human being. Which unknown would Cynthia and her family have to face? Would usual palliative treatments continue to be effective, or would my professional and personal boundaries again be stretched and threat-ened? Cynthia and her family had no choice but to face her uncertain future. I had the privilege and the potential burden of facing it with them.

After an intense, meaningful month at home on hospice, Cynthia's body had deteriorated to the point that she was ready to die. The amount of morphine needed to control her pain now had the effect of sedating her. Each hour she had to choose between enduring severe pain and allowing her consciousness to be clouded. When she was alert she had relentless dry heaves, retching, and hiccoughs. In addition, the smell from her now gaping abdominal wound could not be ignored and was humiliating to Cynthia. She had done the hard work of prepar-ing to die and had said good-bye to all those who had been central to her life. Life as she was now forced to live it had no quality. She looked forward to what the next life might bring.

I felt anxious as I approached Cynthia's house. I knew from our phone conversation just how bad things had gotten and that she was ready to die. But I didn't know how Cynthia hoped to approach the end. The key in my mind was to allow her to die in a way that would allow her to preserve her personhood and would not violate my own values and professional ethics. But our society makes rigid distinctions between methods of easing a patient's death that have little to do with the degree of suffering or the values of the specific patient and doctor. I had promised not to abandon Cynthia and her family, and I was about to discover what that obligation would entail.

Cynthia appeared terribly sick and uncomfortable. The moments of peace and acceptance she had found many times in the last month had disappeared. Her eyes were desperate. She was sad about having to die, but she made it clear to me that her quality of life was intolerable. Several of her options were permissible within current cannons of medical ethics and the law. She was dependent on life-sustaining intravenous infusion of fluids, which she could discontinue. She was also having severe pain and could allow an increase in her morphine infusion to the point of sedation. If death came as an unintended "double effect," so be it, as long as it was not our primary intention. When she asked how long it would take to die, I told her that it would probably take five to ten days, although there were always exceptions. I reassured her that it would not be painful and that she would gradually slip into a very deep sleep. We promised to make every effort to maintain her comfort and dignity throughout the process. She wanted assurance that this method of dying would not be considered a suicide, and I told her that it was both legally and ethically acceptable. She would be "allowed to die" of her underlying disease—that certainly was not suicide.

I asked Cynthia if she was afraid, and she reiterated something she had said in an earlier conversation: that she was more afraid of this phase of dying than of death itself. We had a tearful good-bye. Driving home, I recalled many of my other special patients with whom I had reached this point. I feel that they are being set free from the ordeal that this life has become. Our obligation as medical professionals is to ease their passing as much as possible. It is both wonderful and terrifying. These are experiences I will always carry with me.

My work with Cynthia was not yet complete. The next day, after we stopped the infusion of fluids through her central line, Cynthia felt better than she had in weeks. Taking charge had reinvigorated her, and she decided that she might still have a little of this life in her after all. I let her know that it was fine to restart her central feeding and that we would continue to titrate her morphine drip to maximize her comfort and alertness. All those around her who had begun to let go were a little off balance, but we were willing to see what might happen. Was this the beginning of a miracle? Did we dare hope for such a turnaround? Perhaps we had better take it one day at a time.

Our "miracle" was short-lived. The next day Cynthia's symptoms returned with a vengeance, and she called asking to have her fluids discontinued and her morphine increased. I checked to make sure that she was certain and then made the necessary arrangements. Over the next several days she went into a state of deep somnolence that appeared dreamlike. She clearly was having visions or hallucinations, though they did not appear unpleasant. In her somnolent state she mumbled, "Am I going to get better?" The ray of hope that had sustained her was flickering. "No, I don't think so." She then asked, "Is it time to go?" to which I responded, "Yes, it's time." As she slipped into a coma, she was surrounded by family and friends, who came and sat, sometimes talking softly, other times just being with her. Her parents bid their sad farewell. Tim remained at her side, and a Buddhist priest helped guide her through the transition to her next life. Cynthia died quietly and peacefully, surrounded by loved ones, with her personhood fully intact.

Commentary

1. *Cynthia wanted her doctor to "midwife me through the dying process."* Dying patients need not only competent treatment of their pain and other symptoms but also a broader commitment to work with them throughout the entire process. Even if it reaches into places where the ethical and legal landmarks are unclear, the doctor's obligation is to continue to face the unknown with the patient and his or her family. Health care providers must remain true to their own values, but they should extend themselves to meet the needs of dying persons who may have no acceptable choices. In Cynthia's case, stopping her central fluids and increasing her opioid infusion to the point of sedation at the very end of her life were not good choices, but they were the best of the very restricted options available. They allowed her personhood to remain intact in spite of her body's final disintegration.

The physician's commitment to see the process through no matter what happens can be both liberating and reassuring to patients. Many patients have fears about dying, often based on what they personally have witnessed and on their own values. Because Cynthia was a Buddhist, her fears included being "out of her mind," unable to experience consciousness and to connect with others. She also worried about severe pain and being a burden to her family. She wanted assurance that even if she initially chose an experimental protocol, she could stop aggressive medical treatment later on. She also hoped that if toward the very end she reached a point at which her life was devoid of quality and meaning, she could have help finding death.

Armed with the assurance that she would have a medical partner no matter what her clinical circumstances, Cynthia was able initially to focus on a desperate fight for life and later on to concentrate on enhancing the quality of her remaining life. Severely ill patients and their families look for this degree of commitment from their health care providers. Unfortunately, our current ethical thinking and restrictive laws make it unsafe for physicians to walk with their dying patients when their path enters uncertain terrain. Patients and their families have no choice but to enter these domains; their path is determined in large measure by their underlying disease processes. We must create an ethical, legal, and professional system wherein doctors and other health care providers are encouraged to continue to bring creative solutions to problems even in the most difficult of circumstances.

Although it can have its harrowing moments, working in partnership with patients as they find their way through the transitions from the fight for life to the search for quality of life to their eventual passage into death is a genuine privilege. Each pathway is unique, determined by both the disease process and the profound specificity of the person. Articulate patients like Cynthia can teach us about patients' inner experiences as they pass through this remarkable process. Their stories, rather than abstract debates about public policy, help us to discover what is ultimately important and possible in working with the dying.

2. *How one dies should be consistent with one's values, enhancing rather than diminishing personhood even as the body deteriorates.* Cynthia's dying exemplified a healthy process, filled with heartache, uncertainty, and a series of daunting decisions but carried out in close partnership be-

tween doctor, patient, and family. Cynthia made active choices, but she was guided and challenged by caring professionals. Dying is almost never devoid of suffering and torment. It should, however, also be filled with meaning, connection, and joint decisions by people who care deeply about one another. Cynthia's life and death will be remembered by all those who were a part of it. It was filled with intimacy, generosity, and profound sadness. It reinforced the potential for personal growth and meaning that is possible when people work together to face the tragedy of a premature death.

Dying persons can also feel humiliated or abandoned. Dying inevitably involves a deterioration of the body, but it should not include the disintegration of the person. Cynthia's personhood was most threatened at the beginning and at the end of her dying process. At first she encountered hopelessness and despair as her health and well-being disappeared. Efforts to define the limits of her deterioration seemed fruitless. Once she found an approach that made sense, her personhood was restored, and it remained intact through her subsequent transitions. It was only at the very end, when her quality of life became severely compromised, that her integrity was again threatened. When she was ready to die, and further living had lost its meaning and potential, she and I (as her doctor) were able to find a mutually acceptable solution that allowed her to die peacefully, on terms that she could accept.

Much of the debate about physician-assisted dying has focused on the exact method chosen by doctors and patients who are faced with such untenable dilemmas, minimizing and devaluing the quality of decision making, partnership, and shared meaning they bring to that decision. I believe strongly that the quality of the relationship and commitment brought to these decisions is much more important than abstract judgments about the specific method. Our public policy should encourage doctors to be creative and openly responsive, rather than fearful and secretive, when patients are faced with a bad death. It is our fundamental obligation as physicians not to abandon those patients whom we have committed to care for throughout the dying process.

3. *Hospice can have different meanings at different times in an illness.*

Comfort care, as best exemplified in hospice and palliative care programs, should be considered when suffering is severe and the odds of successful treatment are poor. Too often referrals are made at the last moment, when the patient is at death's door. Such patients and their families are deprived of the opportunity to make peace with one another and with death and to have their medical treatment devoted primarily to relieving suffering. The transition to hospice is often difficult for many patients and families (as well as their physicians); it means giving up on the life-prolonging potential of aggressive medical therapy. For some it is the first time they directly confront their own mortality— a subject often avoided in our culture, even when it stares us in the face.

Although a comfort-oriented approach was appropriately raised early in Cynthia's illness, she initially experienced it as abandonment, an extinguishing of her hope for recovery, which she placed primarily in medical intervention. She felt compelled to try experimental therapy, but she also knew from the outset that there was an alternative approach that would emphasize caring more than curing. Later, after she had experienced a month of what turned out to be futile, invasive medical treatments, comfort care had a radically different meaning for Cynthia. It now offered hope that she could make the most of her remaining time without the added burden of aggressive therapy. There is no formula for how and when to go through these transitions, but hospice care should always be a part of the discussion in the later phases.

References

Caring and Commitment

Council on Scientific Affairs, American Medical Association. Good care of the dying patient. *Journal of the American Medical Association* 275 (1996): 474–78.

Kubler-Ross, E. *On Death and Dying.* New York: Macmillan, 1969.

McCue, J. D. The naturalness of dying. *Journal of the American Medical Association* 273 (1995): 1039–43.

Peabody, F. W. The care of the patient. *New England Journal of Medicine* 88 (1927): 877–82.

Quill, T. E. *Death and Dignity: Making Choices and Taking Charge.* New York: W. W. Norton, 1993.

Quill, T. E., and C. K. Cassel. Nonabandonment: A central obligation for physicians. *Annals of Internal Medicine* 122 (1995): 368–74.

Reich, W. T., and N. S. Jecker. History of the notion of care; historical dimensions of an ethic of care in health care; contemporary ethics of care. In *Encyclopedia of Ethics*, ed. L. C. Becker, 319–44. New York: Garland, 1992.

Wanzer, S. H., S. J. Adelstein, R. E. Cranford, D. D. Federman, E. D. Hook, C. G. Moertel, P. Safar, A. Stone, H. B. Tausig, and J. van Eys. The physician's responsibility toward hopelessly ill patients. *New England Journal of Medicine* 310 (1984): 955–59.

Wanzer, S. H., D. D. Federman, S. J. Adelstein, C. K. Cassel, E. H. Cassem, R. E. Cranford, E. W. Hook, B. Lo, C. G. Moertel, and P. Safar. The physician's responsibility toward hopelessly ill patients: A second look. *New England Journal of Medicine* 320 (1989): 844–49.

Suffering

Angell, M. The quality of mercy. *New England Journal of Medicine* 306 (1982): 98–99.

Cassell, E. J. *The Nature of Suffering and the Goals of Medicine.* New York: Oxford University Press, 1991.

———. The nature of suffering and the goals of medicine. *New England Journal of Medicine* 306 (1992): 639–45.

Delvecchio-Good, M., B. J. Good, C. Schaffer, and S. E. Lind. American oncology and the discourse on hope. *Culture, Medicine and Psychiatry* 14 (1990): 59–79.

Frankl, V. E. *Man's Search for Meaning.* Rev. ed. New York: Washington Square, 1984.

Kapleau, P. (ed). *The Wheel of Death: A Collection of Writings from Zen Buddhist and Other Sources on Death, Rebirth, Dying.* New York: Harper and Row, 1971.

Hospice Referrals

Carlson, R. W., L. Devich, and R. R. Frank. Development of a comprehensive supportive care team for the hopelessly ill on a university hospital medical service. *Journal of the American Medical Association* 259 (1988): 378–83.

Christakis, N. A. Timing of referral of terminally ill patients to an outpatient hospice. *Journal of General Internal Medicine* 9 (1994): 314–20.

Godkin, M. A., J. J. Krant, and J. J. Doster. The impact of hospice care on families. *International Journal of Psychiatry in Medicine* 13 (1983): 153–65.

Mills, M., H. T. Davies, and W. A. Macrae. Care of dying patients in hospital. *British Medical Journal* 309 (1994): 583–86.

Rhymes, J. Hospice care in America. *Journal of the American Medical Association* 264 (1990): 369–72.

Stoddard, S. Hospice in the United States: An overview. *Journal of Palliative Care* 5 (1989): 10–19.

Volicer, L., Y. Rheaume, J. Brown, K. Fabiszewski, and R. Brady. Hospice approach to the treatment of patients with advanced dementia of the Alzheimer type. *Journal of the American Medical Association* 256 (1986): 2210–13.

Wallston, K. A., C. Burger, R. A. Smith, and R. J. Baugher. Comparing the quality of death for hospice and non-hospice cancer patients. *Medical Care* 26 (1988): 177–82.

Chapter 2

Modern Medicine, Distant Drums

IN THE EARLY 1980s a deadly infectious disease that attacked the body's immune system—acquired immunodeficiency syndrome, or AIDS—was first reported. It was initially observed that AIDS primarily affected gay men, but little was known about its causes or transmission. Despite escalating epidemiologic projections, governmental agencies were slow to respond. Our society could not believe that medicine, which had succeeded in overcoming most infectious diseases in the industrialized world, would not readily overcome this threat. The response was also delayed because the majority of the victims were homosexual men, a group toward whom our society is profoundly ambivalent. The number of infected persons was growing exponentially, yet the media, the government, and the medical profession colluded to minimize what was staring them in the face.

Gay men in Rochester, and presumably in most other communities, were scared to death. The 1970s and early 1980s had been a time of relatively free experimentation with sex, and many had participated to one degree or another. The same could be said for heterosexuals, although at the time we falsely believed that the disease would be restricted to homosexual men. Many medical professionals were reluctant to care for these potentially infected men. There appeared to be little effective treatment for the disease, as well as a potential for transmission to the practitioners themselves. Some risk of infectious exposure has traditionally been a part of the medical profession, but this disease was particularly unsettling to those who had been trained in the era of antibiotic effectiveness. Patients in modern times died mainly of cancer and heart disease, and we had little experience of people dying from untreatable infections. Unfortunately, a strong element of homophobia confounded this reluctance. It was not a morally uplifting moment for our society or for our profession.

My practice and several others in Rochester had been identified through the Empty Closet, a gay and lesbian information network, as ones that would accept new, potentially infected patients. Several of our gay patients had already died of rare diseases that, in retrospect, we realized had been complications associated with the earliest cases of AIDS. In 1982 one of our young patients died in the hospital of a mysterious progressive degeneration of his brain. Over a period of six weeks he progressed from walking and talking normally to lying in bed mumbling incoherently, wasting away. He was hallucinating and having seizures much of the time, and he was unable to control his urine or his bowels. He was disintegrating both physically and mentally before our eyes. We seemed powerless to lessen his suffering, much less cure his disease. I remember having nightmares about his illness and wondering about the risk of being exposed to his bodily fluids. Facing such chaotic suffering and having so little to offer, we all felt impotent and at times unnerved.

Robb came into my practice during this uncertain time. He was a large man, solid as a rock from many years in the construction business. He was open and direct about his homosexuality from the outset. He had had many sexual partners in the past but was now in a committed, monogamous relationship with a man named John, which he hoped would last forever. Robb believed that his life would now be settled and satisfying as never before. He had been careful in his sexual contacts in the last few years, but he felt less secure about several of his exposures in the early 1980s. He felt healthy and was able to do physically demanding work. In addition to construction, Robb designed sets and participated in the renovation of GEVA, our nationally recognized regional theater, which had recently moved into a new building. Life was very good, and his future seemed bright.

We talked directly about AIDS and whether he was at risk. At that time there were no reliable screening tests. He had no signs of the disease, although his past sexual exposures put him at risk. We talked about the importance of safe sex and the likelihood that the disease was transmitted through semen or blood. The best preventive measure would be not to expose himself to any new sexual partners and to practice safe sex with John. We seemed to be on the same wavelength. He, much more than I, had been exposed firsthand to the ravages of AIDS, having already lost several friends and acquaintances to the disease (fortunately, none of them had been his sexual partners). We both understood that AIDS was something to be genuinely frightened about, which made minimizing his exposure of the highest importance.

Robb was "out" of the closet with his friends and at his workplace. His parents and sister, however, were another matter. He had visited his family with his "good friend" John, but the depth of their commitment to one another remained unstated. Since his parents had stopped asking about girlfriends and marriage, Robb felt that they were probably aware of his homosexuality. Yet he remained reluctant to risk hurting or alienating his family with an explicit conversation. Since they lived in a rural town in the Northwest, Robb saw no compelling reason to force them to face this aspect of his life. He would maintain this half-secret unless they asked or the perfect opportunity presented itself.

The first few years of my relationship with Robb involved brief contacts concerning work-related injuries: tendinitis from too much hammering, a leg injury from falling off a ladder, a foreign body in his eye, and a dog bite. He then developed bloody diarrhea, which again raised questions about sexually transmitted diseases and AIDS. Although he had had no new sexual exposures, he had been bothered by loose bowel movements intermittently for several years. These symptoms had always disappeared spontaneously, so he had put them out of his mind. In addition to the usual diagnostic considerations such as inflammatory bowel disease, bacterial infections, polyps, and cancer, bloody diarrhea in gay men raises a host of unusual infectious possibilities. We arranged to culture his stool and to examine his lower bowel through a sigmoidoscope. Most of the conditions we were considering were curable or at least controllable with medication.

We revisited the question of testing for human immunodeficiency virus (HIV), the virus that causes AIDS. Reliable testing had become available to determine whether one harbored the virus. I suggested that both Robb and John be tested simultaneously. If they both tested negatively, they could have sex without fear about HIV, provided their relationship remained exclusive. If one or both men tested positively, the situation would be hard to deal with, but treatments were becoming available that altered the course of the disease. Knowing would probably be better than living with constant fear and uncertainty. Robb and John decided to be tested, and they committed to seeing the future together no matter what the outcome.

The test for HIV involves two parts. The first part is a screening test called the EIA (enzyme immunoassay), which picks up more than 99 percent of cases but has some false positives (tests that are abnormal in patients who do not have the disease). Therefore, all positive tests are confirmed by a second test, the Western blot, which eliminates the false positives almost entirely. Only when both tests are positive is the disease confirmed. At that time it took two weeks to get the results for each part of the test. Negative tests usually came back within the first two weeks. It was common knowledge in the gay community that if the results were delayed beyond that point, you were in trouble. This knowledge was not lost on Robb when his results did not return for over four weeks.

Robb had a strong hunch that he would test positively, but there was a frightening finality to actually hearing the bad news. Shaken, he immediately recalled the friends he had lost. Although he wondered whether he would be willing to go through the harsh deterioration that often accompanies the end stages of AIDS, there was no question about his desire to fight the disease. He was willing to do whatever was necessary to stay healthy and functioning. We went over the fact that he had HIV, the virus that causes AIDS, but that it might be many years before he developed the complications that define AIDS. He understood the distinction and hoped to delay the development of AIDS for as long as possible. He wanted to consult with an infectious disease doctor in Rochester who specialized in AIDS and also to explore alternative pathways of activating his spirit in the fight. Since he had a passion for Native American culture, he made an appointment with a therapist who used traditional Native American healing methods in her practice. He left our visit determined and hopeful but also afraid.

John's test came back negative. This was somewhat surprising because he too had been sexually active before their relationship, and he and Robb had had a sexual relationship together for over four years. John felt relieved but also guilty and afraid. Was his test falsely negative, the result of a misleading error in the test that could give him a false sense of security? Would this difference in their HIV status alter their relationship, eroding the trust and love they had developed over the years? What should they do about sex? Must they be cautious about being affectionate with one another? How sick would Robb get, and when would his inevitable deterioration start? Would he be able to handle watching his lover go through the physical and mental deterioration he had witnessed in so many others who had the disease? John and Robb remained clearly committed to one another, but only time would tell whether their feelings of mutual love and connection could be sustained. I reassured them that touching and kissing, as well as routine contact such as sharing towels or utensils, were not dangerous. The disease was not transmitted between family members as long as they avoided contact with the infected party's blood or semen. I emphasized that they must be meticulous about safe sex and recommended that John be tested every six months, just in case.

Robb did not show up for his next visit. Since he had never missed an appointment before, I became concerned. Hearing that one has HIV can be so devastating that a few people commit suicide. Others are plunged into despair, and still others go into complete denial, living their lives as if nothing was wrong. I replayed our previous conversation in my mind and saw no major warning signs. I telephoned Robb. To my relief, he told me that he was making appointments with several AIDS specialists and alternative healers in order to fully explore the medical terrain. I would meet with him when his explorations were complete.

At our next visit we reviewed Robb's strategy. He wanted to pursue a very aggressive biomedical approach being promoted at one of the local AIDS clinics. Every potential new development was being offered to each willing patient. Robb's initial markers of immune function were very good, yet the specialist had already started him on several medications. The potential benefits of giving these drugs at Robb's early stage of illness were based on intuition and underground reports. An extensive information network tracks anything that might be helpful to patients with HIV, and many clinicians recommend each new possibility with hope and enthusiasm. There were downsides to this approach. Patients were repeatedly subjected to "promising" new treatments only to be devastated when they were proven ineffective. In addition to the putting the patient on an emotional roller coaster, more medicine led to an increased potential for toxicity. If side effects occurred, it was often impossible to tell which medication was at fault, so both proven and unproven treatments had to be stopped. In spite of these potential risks, Robb was enthused about an aggressive approach.

Robb initially wanted to receive his HIV-related medical care at the specialty AIDS clinic. He and I would continue to meet in order to review his progress and to explore how he was feeling as a person. I recommended that he avoid unproven therapies unless he was part of a scientific study so that we could eventually learn about their potential effectiveness. Although the temptation was to try everything and anything that could possibly help, we needed to recognize the possibility that more harm than good might result from some of these interventions.

Robb was feeling very alone at this time. John was fully aware of his situation, as were several of his friends. Robb, however, did not want to constantly burden them with his anxieties and concerns. Besides, he needed to talk freely about the effect his diagnosis was having on his closest relationships. His feelings of isolation, fear, and despair were growing, and he needed additional outlets. We discovered several support groups in town for patients with HIV. It was a big step for Robb to contact such a group, for he was not a joiner by nature, but he could always quit if it didn't work out.

This decision was pivotal to the next phase of Robb's illness. He felt an immediate kinship with the other infected members in his group. Every two weeks they met and talked openly about their fear of death, what they had witnessed in other friends, and what they were going through personally. Several members progressed from being HIV-infected to having AIDS and were facing increasingly severe complications. Seeing his infected friends deteriorate was frightening, but it also helped Robb grasp his own uncertain future. Robb found that he could talk very openly with the members of this group, exploring his fears and hopes without having to justify or protect anyone. The bonds he forged in the group helped sustain him through to the end of his illness.

One of the major difficulties Robb was struggling with was what to tell his parents. His parents had fully accepted John as his "friend," yet he still had not openly discussed his homosexuality with them. He eventually shared the details of his life and his diagnosis with his sister. Although she had strongly suspected that he was gay, the news about his infection still came as a shock. Robb and his sister explored the pros and cons of protecting their parents from the information. By not telling them, they allowed their parents to maintain the illusion that their son was not gay, much less HIV infected. On the other hand, it was likely that his parents knew he was gay and had unstated fears about his being HIV-positive that could not be voiced without violating their family secret. The net effect of this secret was to impair direct communication whenever they were together. When and if he became sicker in the future, they would be unprepared.

Robb finally shared the details of his illness and the nature of his relationship with John with his parents. Although they were initially overwhelmed, they could not have been more accepting and supportive. They had suspected all along he was gay but were waiting for him to bring it out into the open. His parents genuinely liked John and immediately accepted him even more fully into their family. They had had no previous experience with these things, coming from a generation that kept potentially embarrassing or controversial problems hidden.

Nonetheless, they were glad that Robb had told them, and they became central players in the web of support that Robb was weaving.

For the HIV-positive individual, every ache, pain, or fever may be a harbinger of life-threatening illness. Interpreting these sensations is therefore a formidable challenge, because the usual background symptoms that affect us all also occur in those with HIV. Is this cough and fever the sign of a simple cold that is running through the community, or is it the beginning of an opportunistic, potentially life-threatening pneumonia because of my suppressed immune system? Is the rash on my arm an allergic reaction to poison ivy, or is it the first sign of Kaposi's sarcoma, an unusual cancer with a particular predilection to AIDS patients? The answers to these questions are not immediately obvious to patients with HIV, because they are at increased risk for many unusual diseases. Yet they are also still subject to the aches and pains of everyday life.

In addition, we regularly monitor the function of the immune system for patients with HIV by checking their CD4 count. When the CD4 count falls below 200, the risk of complications is increased and more prophylactic treatments are indicated. There is considerable background variation in CD4 counts in healthy patients as well as those with HIV. Therefore, one often doesn't know whether the drop that periodically occurs in the background is a sign of increasing vulnerability or a normal test variation. If one is prone to anxiety, this variation can drive one crazy. Eventually, HIV-infected patients either make peace with this background noise—both of test fluctuations and of common symptoms—or else live every day in constant fear.

Robb was extremely anxious at first. Since it was such a new disease, how could we be sure that we were not overlooking something? The answer was that we couldn't be 100 percent sure, but if he lived each moment in fear, the quality of his life would suffer. Robb needed to seek medical attention for problems that seemed serious or progressive or were not resolving in the normal course of events. Yet, if one visits enough doctors about minor concerns, there is considerable risk of medical overtreatment. We agreed to meet regularly so that we could review his experiences and I could answer questions. If he had pressing concerns between appointments, he could call me to discuss whether he needed to be seen. The members of his support group shared similar struggles in coping with their disease: How could they be vigilant without being completely paranoid? Where could they get the best medical care when so little was known about the disease? How could they live a full life with a death threat hanging over their heads? How should they cope with family and friends who were now treating them differently?

Robb did very well over the next two years. He became an expert about his disease and was a resource for himself and others. He continued his construction job and was busy doing the design work that he loved on the side. He generally felt well, and he was able to put his worries about his future out of his mind most of the time. He allowed them to surface mainly in the biweekly meetings of his support group and during doctor's visits, which averaged once per month. He took full advantage of his six weeks of vacation each year and traveled extensively with John to places they had always wanted to visit. John had adjusted reasonably well to Robb's illness and had become his stalwart support. Together, they succeeded in living life fully in the present.

Although Robb continued to feel well, his CD4 count began to drop. As a result, he was put on more and more medication by his AIDS specialist in an attempt to forestall the inevitable. Combination therapy using several drugs simultaneously to fight the virus has become the standard of care in recent years, although many of the medicines Robb was initially taking have been proven ineffective. Robb started feeling uncomfortable about all the medication (eight different medicines, thirty-six doses per day, plus one inhalation treatment per month). We met to discuss which ones might be eliminated. His CD4 count had fallen below 200, so his risk of developing opportunistic infections was definitely increased. The medical indication for preventive treatment against opportunistic infection was now clear, as was the need for medicine to fight the HIV virus. After I gave Robb my recommendations about eliminating some of his nonessential medications, he made an appointment to discuss this with his AIDS specialist.

Before that appointment Robb developed hives, a rash indicative of a systemic allergic reaction. Since they were most likely a side effect of his medications, we had to discontinue all of them since we did not know which one was the culprit. The hives disappeared almost immediately. We then gradually restarted the essential medications and made substitutions for those most commonly associated with allergic reactions. We cut the number of medications he was taking from eight to four, and we cut his total daily doses down to sixteen per day. He again felt better, but his CD4 count was now under 100. Trouble was on the way, but we did not know when or in what form.

Robb had another year of good health. Having achieved a peace with his vulnerability, he had succeeded in living one day at a time. He felt well mentally and remained fully active physically. At one of our routine meetings he showed me a purplish lesion on his thigh. It was slightly raised and firm, and there had been no trauma. I immediately recognized it as Kaposi's sarcoma. Robb also had suspected this, so my confirmation came as no surprise. The manifestations of Kaposi's sarcoma can range from a relatively minor skin lesion of no clinical consequence to an invasive condition that spreads throughout the body. Chemotherapy and radiation are only marginally effective, and surgery does not work. We elected to take a wait-and-see approach, hoping that his Kaposi's sarcoma would be inconsequential. I consulted several experienced medical oncologists; they were pessimistic about the effect of chemotherapy but would try it if Robb's disease progressed.

Unfortunately, Robb's Kaposi's sarcoma was very aggressive. He returned one month later with several new lesions on his thigh, swollen lymph glands in his groin, and swelling in his feet. For Robb this progression marked a clear transition in his illness. For the first time, Robb was having difficulty doing his job because of his physical limitations. His leg was swollen and sore, and work exhausted him. He didn't know how much time he had left or how much quality his life would have, but he did not want to spend every ounce of his spare energy working. Robb had been reluctant to apply for Social Security disability payments, but he was now ready to make this transition. He definitely met the requirements; it was simply a matter of completing the paperwork. Yet work had been a defining theme in Robb's life since he was a teenager. What would take the place of the meaning and focus that it had provided?

Robb then discovered AIDS Mastery, a program in the Rochester community for HIV-infected patients, their families, and health care providers devoted to a full understanding of the disease. This program was to play a central role in the last phase of Robb's life. In spite of his declining physical abilities, he tried to achieve "mastery" of his illness. His education was both medical and personal, including a series of weekend encounter groups. There were no taboos in these discussions, as participants integrated biological, psychological, and social perspectives. The spiritual implications were also explored, and Robb's affinity to Native American traditions was given full expression. He met with a woman named Dixie, who guided him in a deeper exploration of Native American spirituality. Death was not necessarily something to be feared but an opportunity to be reconnected with one's ancestors—a coming together of past and future, a different plane of existence. Robb found the universal connection to other living things, the land, and his personal history very comforting. The ritual chants, drumming, guided imagery, and meditation helped keep meaning in his life and provided respite from his losses. His spiritual life blossomed as his body was deteriorating.

Robb began chemotherapy with bleomycin and vincristine as his Kaposi's sarcoma continued its relentless progression. The lesions seemed to shrink, and the swelling in his legs decreased. Unfortunately, his blood counts also went down, limiting the amount of chemotherapy he could receive. Several especially troubling spots were treated with brief courses of radiation therapy. We were in no way curing the disease, but perhaps we could control it for a time.

In the background, many of Robb's friends and acquaintances were dying. He had been to so many funerals that it became difficult to grieve or even to engage in the losses of others. For Robb, how people died took on new meaning and urgency. The extremes of these journeys ranged from dying in the hospital, emaciated and demented after trying every conceivable medical avenue, to making a preemptive strike by overdosing with barbiturates at the first sign of deterioration. Robb did not want either of these extremes, but he did want to be given as much leeway as possible in the middle ground. He knew that if he lost the capacity to make decisions for himself, he wanted comfort measures only and absolutely no life-prolonging treatments. Robb requested that John become his health care proxy. He felt certain that John could best represent his values and wishes in the event that he could not articulate them himself. Robb's parents might be too reluctant to let go of their son. For Robb, this would have been the worst possible outcome. Although signing his advance directive was reassuring to him, it was another indication of his inevitable decline.

The next six months were not easy for Robb. He developed vertigo, a sensation that is usually indicative of a mild inner-ear problem but is also a potential sign of brain deterioration in a patient with AIDS. An extensive search for an underlying brain lesion showed no complications; it was probably labyrinthitis, a common abnormality of the inner ear that resolves spontaneously. Robb's vertigo gradually disappeared, but his vulnerability was increasing. The Kaposi's sarcoma became less and less responsive to chemotherapy, and we repeatedly had to artificially stimulate his bone marrow to help him manufacture enough white blood cells. Experimental treatment with interferon was the next possibility, but we were rapidly running out of options. The first scheduled treatment with interferon was postponed until after Robb had visited family and friends on the West Coast. We always tried to schedule his treatments and appointments so that they didn't interfere with travel or other special events. The Kaposi's sarcoma limited his quality of life but was not in itself life threatening. If his time was to be limited, we didn't want him to miss the opportunity for experiences that enhanced the quality of his remaining time.

Robb and John had a good trip to the West Coast. All of his family was present for a reunion. Although their conversations generally avoided his illness, Robb was obviously not as robust and optimistic as he had been in the past. Everyone sensed that their time together was precious. Toward the end of the visit, Robb developed a low-grade fever and had mild difficulty in breathing. He cut his visit short by a week and returned to Rochester. By the time he was on the plane he was having shaking chills, high fever, and increasing shortness of breath. He called me from the airport, and I arranged to meet him in the emergency department. Robb had always wanted to avoid the hospital. He had seen too much when he visited his friends there. I knew that he must be very sick if he was agreeing to go.

Robb was indeed severely ill when I saw him in the emergency room. He had bilateral pneumonia, a very low white blood cell count, and a low oxygen level. We treated him for both common bacterial pneumonias and pneumocystis carinii (PCP), a protozoa that frequently causes lung infections in patients with AIDS. He was given a breathing mask to increase oxygen delivery and injections to stimulate his white blood cells. Arrangements were made to use a tube to directly sample the cells in his lungs (bronchoscopy), since very unusual organisms can affect the lungs of patients with AIDS. The bronchoscopy confirmed PCP, and his antibiotic coverage was adjusted. Corticosteroids were added, since they had been shown to be of benefit to patients with this severe infection. We would now wait and hope that the medicine worked its magic.

Robb had never been a hospital patient. He suffered extreme discomfort from shortness of breath, shaking chills, repeated blood tests, and a harsh, painful cough. He also found the lack of control and the sheer numbers of people who had some influence over his well-being to be terrifying. The interns and residents often communicated slightly different information from the infectious disease specialist, which in turn differed subtly from what I was telling him. He would ask each member of the health care team how he was doing, and every small discrepancy added to his anxiety. The members of the health care team eventually contracted with Robb to have all information flow through me, as his primary physician. We agreed to seek a consensus whenever possible before communicating new information.

Robb was aware that his repeated requests for additional information were a subterfuge for his real fear, namely, that this was the beginning of the steep downhill slide toward his death. Having witnessed harsh deaths in friends who had had AIDS, Robb was now much more afraid of dying badly than he was of death itself. Still, Robb was not ready to die if it could be prevented. Fortunately, he was gradually improving. This would likely be his closest scrape so far, but he had also seen some friends come back from hospitalization and return to a life filled with quality. He remained frightened but cautiously optimistic.

One week later Robb suddenly deteriorated. His shortness of breath increased dramatically, and his oxygen level dropped abruptly. A repeat chest x-ray was described as a "snowstorm." Robb's life was now truly threatened. The potential causes of his abrupt decline included a resistant form of PCP, a second opportunistic infection, and adult respiratory distress syndrome (a complication of severe lung injury in which the membranes become very porous and fluid accumulates). Robb was transferred to our intensive care unit, and plans were initiated to temporarily put him on a mechanical breathing machine. We were relatively confident that we could pull him through; there was no doubt about how to proceed from a medical point of view.

I went to the intensive care unit to explain the next steps to Robb. John was at his side. They both appeared frightened, although each stayed composed for the other's sake. I started with a simplified version about what to expect, knowing we had to act relatively quickly because of Robb's rapidly deteriorating medical condition. There was not enough time to contemplate all the options in detail or to fully inform them.

Robb immediately interrupted me: "Tim, what is the point?" he asked.

I wondered where this was going. Given his medically critical condition, a lengthy discussion was impossible. "What do you mean?"

"I mean where is this all going?" Robb reiterated.

I responded literally, to the present crisis. "We hope you will be on the ventilator for only a few days, until we get the infection identified and treated. Once that occurs, we hope you will improve and return to the life you had been living."

"I don't like the way I have been living, and I can only see things getting worse. If all I had was this pneumonia, I'd say go ahead. You can cure me from this pneumonia, but you can't cure my cancer or my AIDS. I don't want to waste away like I've seen all my friends."

I tried to convince Robb otherwise. I was not mentally prepared for this conversation. So much was riding on it, and there was no time for deep reflection and second thoughts. "You might recover and get a lot of good-quality time. I would hate to have you lose that time when this might be a readily reversible problem."

"I've had a lot of time to think while I have been in the hospital, and I have had enough. I just don't see the point of enduring more Hell right now so that I can experience further deterioration in the future."

"But we don't know for certain what the future will bring, and I promise that we will face what has to be faced together. I will do my best to not have you suffer unnecessarily. Besides, you could try going on the ventilator, and if it didn't seem to be working, or you hate it, we could stop at any time."

"I've thought about it a lot, and I want to stop now."

"Are you sure? Because there is a good chance that we can turn this around."

"It is the only path that makes any sense to me."

I involved John in the conversation. He repeated all the arguments for Robb to keep going, and Robb consistently countered each one. Robb was much further along in his thinking than either of us. John tried to convince Robb that he needed him and that life would be empty for him without Robb. But, as always, John would completely support Robb's decision.

"Robb, you need to know that you will likely die without the ventilator," I pleaded, hoping he would change his mind.

"I know that. I am as ready as I am going to be," Robb replied.

"If you choose not to go on the breathing machine, we can either continue all other treatments and testing, hoping they will begin to work and pull you through, or we can shift to only using treatments to keep you comfortable. In that case, we will give you morphine for your shortness of breath if it becomes uncomfortable, and we will stop all treatments that are not directly connected to your immediate comfort. You will assuredly die with this approach, but we can minimize your suffering in the process."

Robb responded, "I am ready to die, and I don't want to suffer any more."

I left the room shaken by the conversation. I had gone in steeled for a medical battle complete with the use of advanced medical technology, and I left trying to make the abrupt transition to comfort care. I often take the lead in this transition, but this time the shift had been initiated by Robb. Most of my other patients with AIDS had been through multiple difficult hospitalizations, often dying in the midst of a heroic medical battle, without taking full advantage of comfort-oriented care. Robb was making the transition during his first major hospital crisis. Yet to say that he had not suffered enough would be so far from the truth as to be absurd. His decision did give added perspective about just how much anguish some people are willing to endure and how it is impossible to know one's capacity in advance. As I stepped back and reflected, it made perfect sense for Robb to face this crisis with clarity and courage, sensing the opportunity for a dignified exit in order to avoid the extremes of deterioration he had witnessed in others.

I reported my conversation with Robb to the staff, who were poised to begin their invasive interventions. Compared with many patients who pass through the intensive care unit toward the end of their lives, Robb was relatively intact. He was young and had never been hospitalized before. He would probably respond to our interventions at least this time. The staff had encountered many AIDS patients who had survived repeated trips through the intensive care unit before finally succumbing to their illness. Yet they knew only too well what Robb's future held, and they respected his decision.

We decided that Robb could best be cared for on the regular medical floor, where he had originally been admitted and where everybody knew him. Even though "nothing was going to be done" to prolong his life from a purely biomedical point of view, the medical residents got reinvolved so that they could help to provide comfort and support. We agreed to discontinue his antibiotics and lab work. Robb's primary discomforts were shortness of breath and coughing, both of which could be treated with an intravenous infusion of morphine. Although morphine is very effective in relieving these symptoms, it can also depress respirations and contribute to an earlier death. Having prescribed morphine under similar circumstances many times as a primary care physician and a hospice medical director, I was comfortable with its inherent ambiguity. For medical residents, whose main clinical training is in the all-out fight for life, using morphine for this purpose was much more of a struggle. We agreed that given Robb's goals and clinical circumstances, our foremost obligation was to relieve his suffering. Robb's death was inevitable. Allowing him to experience severe symptoms of suffocation that could end only in his death was morally and professionally unacceptable. With my reassurance and support, the medical residents were able to order liberal amounts of morphine and promise Robb it would be increased as much as necessary to keep him comfortable. The residents learned firsthand from Robb about allowing patients to take charge in the face of adversity.

Robb's final hours in the hospital were memorable for all those who were fortunate enough to be working that night. A former therapist from the AIDS Mastery program tried to convince him to reconsider aggressive treatment but finally accepted Robb's clear refusal. John remained steadfastly at his side, and Dixie, his friend with experience in Native American rituals, was invited to join them. Robb was initially very alert and talkative. He and John reviewed their life together and speculated about what Robb's next life might be like. The poking, prodding, and monitoring that usually characterizes death in twentieth-century America were replaced by chanting, drumming, and praying. For a brief moment the medical floor was transported to a time, a place, and a culture in which death was accepted and sometimes even welcomed. Robb's morphine infusion was gradually increased over the evening when his shortness of breath increased. He peacefully slipped into a coma and died, with drums receding in the background.

Commentary

1. *Moments of truth in clinical decision making often present themselves with unanticipated suddenness.* I have always been a staunch advocate of patients' rights to refuse or discontinue potentially life-sustaining treatment, but I was unprepared for the transition at the end of Robb's life. A striking gap often exists between abstract principles and clinical reality. Perhaps I was reluctant because Robb appeared so young and healthy. Maybe I felt too close to him to let go so suddenly. My prior experience with many other AIDS patients had been that they usually hung onto life until the last possible moment, often enduring considerable suffering in the process. Furthermore, most decisions to stop treatment are made over more time, contemplated, considered, and then reconsidered. This decision was unexpected at the time, coming when I was in the midst of nurturing Robb through his first hospitalization for a potentially treatable infection. I had anticipated that these issues might emerge after he left the hospital, when we both would have more time and perspective to reflect.

We were not allowed this luxury. The question was posed, and we had to make a decision between two bad choices. On the one hand, he could go onto the ventilator and hope to recover and then, if he was lucky, go home and face what had to be faced. On the other hand, he could refuse to go onto the ventilator and likely die in a matter of hours. In our conversation, so compressed in time, Robb had clearly chosen the latter course. He understood his condition and the consequences of his decision. Once it was fully articulated and explored, overriding it was out of the question.

The chanting and drums that accompanied Robb's peaceful departure from this life provided a rich and resonant contrast to breathing machines, monitors, and cardiopulmonary resuscitation in an intensive care unit. Life's final chapter in modern medical facilities often ends in the chaos of a futile fight for life, with harsh chest compressions, electric shocks to the heart, and tubes down the throat. If how one leaves this world has any bearing on how one enters the next, we should probably be much more circumspect about how we treat our dying. Robb's death was peaceful and uplifting, and we all felt privileged to be a part of it.

2. *Medical students and residents rarely get to work closely with patients as they make the transition from aggressive, life-prolonging treatment to a comfort-oriented approach.* We would never allow medical students and residents to complete their training without knowing how to perform cardiopulmonary resuscitation, but most current graduates do not know the basics of how to relieve pain and address the suffering of the terminally ill. Our duty to relieve human suffering must be elevated to the same level as our mandate to fight for life, in both training and practice. Many times, patients treated with a comfort-oriented approach are considered to be good "material" for teaching the important skills of diagnosis and treatment. They are often "uncovered" (no longer seen by students and residents) when they make the transition to palliative care. "Why see them if we are not going to do anything?" is the way the question is often posed. Thus, trainees rarely learn the skills needed to make the transition to comfort care, nor do they learn how to relieve symptoms and promote personal contact and spiritual growth once it is acknowledged that the patient is dying.

Keeping trainees involved with articulate patients like Robb does more to educate them about palliative care than most didactic lectures and readings. Actually having to prescribe morphine to someone who is dying of respiratory failure forces the clinician to confront the "double effect" in all its complexity. Morphine is necessary to prevent the sensation of suffocation, one of the most devastating symptoms to which the terminally ill are subjected. Yet, paradoxically, it can also indirectly contribute to death by suppressing respirations. Although this is not the primary intention, it *feels* as though we are directly contributing to death. Until one has thought through, experienced, and felt this process, one may be reluctant to prescribe adequate analgesia to dying patients. These and many other complex challenges in caring for the dying should be worked through under careful supervision in training so that the next generation of physicians will be more skilled and less frightened about fulfilling their obligation to care for the dying.

3. *HIV-infected patients, through their activism and leadership, have helped change the practice of medicine.* Many individuals and groups have been very vocal in their advocacy for more research and for shortening the time needed for clinical trials. With so many dying, and so little effective treatment, the need for a speedy, responsive process for developing new treatments is compelling. Substantial changes in the approval process for new drugs have occurred as a result of the work of AIDS advocacy groups. This activism has also contributed to an evolution in the doctor-patient relationship from an authoritarian model to one based on partnership and collaboration. In this relationship, the patient's ideas and initiatives are an essential part of the decision-making equation. From the beginning, Robb was an active participant in all aspects of his illness. He most clearly took the lead at the end and was therefore able to die in a way that integrated his values and wishes. His choice was determined to some degree by his clinical situation but mostly by his willingness to look at his future objectively and face his inevitable demise. Having witnessed bad deaths, Robb felt that dying now was better than facing a future in which he might be subjected to further losses and potential humiliations. He wanted to die while his personhood remained intact.

Many patients with HIV and AIDS have seen too much death. Witnessing a friend's dying badly of AIDS dementia makes one genuinely frightened about the future and unwilling to accept the false reassurance that the medical profession can always relieve suffering. Many HIV-infected patients want to live as long as their life can have meaning and dignity, but they want to avoid humiliation at the end if their suffering can only be relieved by death. Rather than wait for the medical and legal professions to decide how they should be "allowed to die," even under the most devastating of circumstances, AIDS activists have formed informal networks whereby patients can get the assistance they need. Many residential hospices devoted exclusively to AIDS patients have been developed outside the traditional medical care system, supported financially by private fund-raising and clinically by a rich matrix of volunteers. Activists on both sides of the continent have also found ways to obtain barbiturates as a last resort for their friends in need. Surrounded by so much illness and death, one's willingness to wait for our society to comprehend the reality faced by patients dying with AIDS is limited.

References

Moments of Truth

Annas, G. J. Informed consent, cancer and truth in prognosis. *New England Journal of Medicine* 330 (1994): 223–25.

Lo, B. Improving care near the end of life: Why is it so hard? *Journal of the American Medical Association* 274 (1995): 1634–36.

Miyaji, N. The power of compassion: Truth-telling among American doctors in the care of dying patients. *Social Science and Medicine* 36 (1993): 249–64.

Pellegrino, E. D. Is truth telling to the patient a cultural artifact? *Journal of the American Medical Association* 268 (1992): 1734–35.

Surbone, A. Truth telling to the patient. *Journal of the American Medical Association* 268 (1992): 1661–62.

Teaching about Death and Dying

American Board of Internal Medicine. *Caring for the Dying—Identification and Promotion of Clinical Competency: Educational Resource Document.* Philadelphia, 1996.

Artiss, K. L., and A. S. Levine. Doctor-patient relation in severe illness: A seminar for oncology fellows. *New England Journal of Medicine* 288 (1973): 1210–14.

Billings, J. A. Medical education for hospice care: A selected bibliography with brief annotations. *Hospice Journal* 9 (1993): 69–83.

Knight, C. F., P. F. Knight, M. H. Gellula, and G. H. Holman. Training our future physicians: A hospice rotation for medical students. *American Journal of Hospice and Palliative Care* 9 (1992): 23–28.

Mermann, A. C., D. B. Gunn, and G. E. Dickinson. Learning to care for the dying: A survey of medical schools and a model course. *Academic Medicine* 66 (1991): 35–38.

Rappaport, W., and D. Witzke. Education about death and dying during the clinical years of medical school. *Surgery* 113 (1993): 163–65.

AIDS

Aoun, H. From the eye of the storm, with the eyes of a physician. *Annals of Internal Medicine* 116 (1991): 335–38.

Angell, M. A dual approach to the AIDS epidemic. *New England Journal of Medicine* 324 (1991): 1498–1500.

Buehler, J. W., and J. W. Ward. A new definition for AIDS surveillance. *Annals of Internal Medicine* 118 (1993): 390–92.

Copeland, A. R. Suicide among AIDS patients. *Medicine, Science and the Law* 33 (1993): 21–28.

Grey, M. R. Syphilis and AIDS in Belle Glade, Florida, 1942 and 1992. *Annals of Internal Medicine* 116 (1992): 329–34.

Sontag, S. *Illness as Metaphor.* New York: Doubleday, 1990.

U.S. Public Health Service/Infectious Diseases Society of America. USPHS/IDSA guidelines for the prevention of opportunistic infections in persons infected with human immunodeficiency virus: A summary. *Annals of Internal Medicine* 124 (1996): 349–68.

Chapter 3

"Do You Still Love Me?"

W E CAME TO know each other in spite of many obstacles. Mrs. Martinez spoke very little English and I spoke almost no Spanish. One of her daughters, who was fluent in both languages, served as a translator. Unfortunately, her translations often digressed into mother-daughter diatribes in Spanish that I had no way of understanding or participating in. The summaries of these heated conversations would be brief comments such as "It's okay" or "She understands." Her daughter would frequently come to the office visits intoxicated, further confounding our already substantial communication problems. Mrs. Martinez herself had been a heavy drinker and a smoker. She had quit drinking after developing cirrhosis of the liver and bleeding esophageal varices ten years previously, and she had stopped smoking at about the same time because of repeated pulmonary infections and asthma. Most of her early visits revolved around recurrent respiratory problems.

In spite of the many barriers between us, Mrs. Martinez always seemed to be someone special. She had a twinkle in her eye, a faint smile, and a raised eyebrow that would nonverbally communicate her exasperation with her daughter's translations and her desire for more direct contact. Unfortunately, the odds of our coming to know each other personally were very poor. The differences between our worlds seemed too great to bridge successfully.

We continued to have relatively limited, unsatisfying appointments about twice a year for the first three years of our relationship. Bronchitis, pneumonia, a laceration, and indigestion—medical transactions involving little explicit personal exchange. This changed when her husband had a heart attack and was admitted to the coronary care unit under my care. He had diabetes and atherosclerosis. His heart attack was extensive, and his heart began to fail as a pump. Fluid was backing up in his lungs, and he would likely die if we did not intervene aggressively. A coronary arteriogram showed blocked arteries that could be corrected with surgery. There were risks in all directions, but the odds of his dying would be considerably less with surgery than without it; there were no guarantees and no easy choices. Mr. Martinez feared surgery, and he wanted his family to help him make the decision. We were again working through intermediaries, but this time a professional translator was used.

The Martinez family meetings were raucous affairs, a chaotic mix of intense emotional expression and multiple simultaneous conversations in English and Spanish. Five children, four spouses, and ten grandchildren were usually present. The oldest sons emerged as the central decision makers. Fortunately, they were both fluent in English and Spanish. They carefully listened to the medical information. Although the best odds were with surgery, it was not without considerable risk. They talked with their father for a long time in Spanish, the rest of the family hanging on every word. Mr. Martinez reluctantly consented to the surgery. Throughout the discussion Mrs. Martinez listened intently in the background, saying nothing but communicating everything with her tear-filled eyes. She did not participate in the exchange of words, but at each juncture her sons and her husband looked to her for approval.

I asked the oldest son how his father had reached his decision. He described Mr. Martinez's fear about leaving his wife. They had been constant companions for the past forty years. Even when he was in the hospital she would spend the night in the chair near his bed, in part as a support but also because separation was painful and frightening. Mr. Martinez was more fearful of abandoning his wife than he was of dying. His consent for surgery was fully informed, but he went into it with a distinct feeling that he would not survive. I felt unsettled about his decision, but further procrastination would have put him at even more risk. Fear seemed to dominate hope; we were all quietly on edge.

The news from the operating room could not have been worse.

Mr. Martinez's bypass surgery was initially uneventful, but the surgeons were unable to "restart" his heart after the procedure. He died on the operating table after an hour-long effort at cardiopulmonary resuscitation. His family was summoned to a "quiet room." They knew something had gone wrong. When they heard the news, they were overcome with guilt and grief. They pleaded to God with agonizing screams. Several people fainted, others pounded the walls, and still others hugged one another as they sobbed unabashedly. Although the scene appeared chaotic and somewhat frightening to me (a few tears discretely wiped away and a gentle hug are more the norm from my cultural perspective), there was a wonder and ritual to the process. Those who weren't crying were integrated in spite of their reticence, and those who needed to rage were allowed to do so. The pain was palpable, out in the open; responses were loud, irrational, overwhelming, and fully accepted. Although the sons eventually wanted to hear exactly what had happened in the operating room, their belief in the power of God was much more central to understanding this tragedy than the impotence of the medical profession. The language of their grief was Spanish, but there was no need for translation to understand the meaning and depth of their pain.

As the shock and emotion began to dissipate, the family turned their attention to their mother. She had not been alone in forty years. Where would she go from here, and with whom? We agreed that for the short term she would stay with one of her daughters. Within a day I got a call saying that Mrs. Martinez couldn't sleep, was overwhelmed by anxiety, and was driving everybody crazy. I sent her a prescription for antianxiety medication and made arrangements for an office visit. She came in with her daughter, who was once again intoxicated. I could not determine who was speaking for whom or who needed treatment more. During this visit I learned that Mrs. Martinez could speak much more English that I had realized. I began to bypass her daughter and speak with Mrs. Martinez directly. She spoke tearfully about her fear of living alone, but she also described how her family was suffocating her with their oversolicitousness. We agreed that she would stay with her daughter for another week and then return to her own home. An hour-long complete physical exam was set up for a few weeks later.

Mrs. Martinez came by herself to her next appointment, and several details of her life story were filled in. She was the only surviving member in her generation of eight children. The "baby" of the family, she had always received special treatment. Most of her siblings had died of cancer; she had seen several of them die painful deaths. Mrs. Martinez was terrified of death, but she was even more frightened of dying in pain and out of control, as several of her relatives had. Mrs. Martinez lamented her husband's death, but she found some solace in the fact that his death had involved so little pain and suffering. In the past, caring for her husband had been her main reason for living. She had monitored his sugars, his diet, and his medicine, spending much of her life anticipating and fulfilling his every need. She was not sure that she could keep going without him. Her family discouraged her from expressing these painful feelings. Not being able to share her grief made it even more isolating and extreme. When we explored the prospect of returning to her home, I discovered she had several widowed women friends in her apartment complex with whom she felt very connected. They had found a way to survive the loss of their husbands. Perhaps in this new phase of her life she would not be as isolated as she had thought.

Mrs. Martinez's return home went better than anyone expected. She played cards and gossiped with her new friends nightly, and her family soon complained that she was never home. Yet the transition was not always easy. At times she felt overwhelmed by fear and aloneness. She made several visits to the emergency department because of chest pain, which was probably attributable more to her "broken heart" and her fear of dying than to a physiological heart disease. Over the next year Mrs. Martinez's feelings of well-being and competence increased gradually. She even explored the idea of taking driving lessons for the first time, at age seventy-five. A strong feeling of connection was developing between us, and I began to look forward to our visits as a time when something special often happened.

Two years later, blossoming as a person, Mrs. Martinez noted an ulcer in the back of her throat. She had been a heavy smoker in the past, and she had lost one sibling to oral cancer. The writing was on the wall. She knew how challenging the treatment of oral cancer, which included deforming surgery and radiation that often forestalled but did not always prevent a difficult death, could be. "Could it be cancer?" she asked. Should I tell her the truth or protect her? How much did she really want to know? How much should I involve her family? "Yes, it could be, but there is no way to know without a biopsy." I waited, letting her control the flow and depth of information. Mrs. Martinez did not want to know more at that time, but she thought I should talk to her sons.

Cultural differences between doctor and patient may create unanticipated misconceptions, so the necessity of establishing explicit understanding and shared meaning is essential. "What would it mean to you if the ulcer is a cancer?" I asked.

"I would be scared to death, for I saw my older sister die of mouth cancer, and it was horrible."

"I hope that it is not. But if it is, we have better ways of dealing with cancer now that can usually prevent such 'horrible' problems. Whatever it is, we will figure out what to do together."

Partially reassured, Mrs. Martinez was scheduled for a biopsy. At home her thoughts were dominated by mutilation, suffering, and death. Trying to minimize the agony of waiting, we scheduled her biopsy as quickly as possible. A follow-up appointment was scheduled for several days later. The results showed a *necrotizing sialometaplasia*. Having never seen or heard of this entity, I rapidly looked it up, then called the pathologist. It was a benign, self-limited condition of unknown cause! I breathed a loud sigh of relief and looked forward to our visit later that day. The dread I had been feeling lifted.

This joyous news reinforced Mrs. Martinez's feeling that her personal evolution and growth since her husband's death had been in the right direction. Her new self-assertiveness and confidence would not be undermined, and the future held the potential for even more self-expression. Mrs. Martinez was so young at heart that I wondered aloud if she might be ready to share her life with a new partner. She allowed that this was not out of the question but then said that she was going to save herself only for me. Our feelings of connection and affection were explicit and in the open. We ended our visit with a kiss and a hug, expressions of our shared joy about the medical bullet that she had just dodged, her increasing growth as an independent person, and our special feelings for one another.

Over the next three years I saw Mrs. Martinez about three times a year, mainly to treat respiratory infections. The visits were also opportunities for her to give voice to fears about a heart attack, cancer, and death. I encouraged her to speak freely about these matters and to share them with me since her family discouraged discussion of such things. I promised to take her concerns seriously and to keep a vigilant watch for problems without subjecting her to repeated, unnecessary testing. Our visits always began with a kiss and ended with a hug, a ritual to which we both looked forward. Mrs. Martinez's visits were a bright spot in my day. She now came to her appointments alone, so our communication was unencumbered by a translator. Her English was more than sufficient for us to discuss most medical matters. Although she remained fearful about the future, my reassurances about her health were always rejoined by a comment from Mrs. Martinez about the importance of our relationship to her.

In 1988, seven years after our initial encounter and four years after her husband's death, Mrs. Martinez developed black, tarry stools, a sign of bleeding from her stomach. She feared that this was the beginning of the end. However, she had had similar stomach bleeding from her liver cirrhosis fifteen years earlier, so she was not as anxious as she might otherwise have been. An x-ray of her stomach showed a large gastric mass. It looked like cancer, but there were some peculiar features. "Is it cancer?" she asked. "It may be," I told her, "although we are not sure." The family gathered to explore the approach. We had all been through this before. "Before you become too alarmed," I told them, "we have arranged for a look through a tube into her stomach to see what it is." Surprisingly, the look in her stomach showed swollen veins from her liver cirrhosis as the probable source of her bleeding. The mass could not be seen. It was probably beneath the inner surface of the stomach. We needed to talk about surgery for both diagnosis and treatment.

Mrs. Martinez dreaded the prospect of surgery. She immediately thought of her husband, dying on the operating table. Could it happen to her? We talked about the differences between his surgery and hers. The odds were good that her tumor was curable, provided it could be removed completely. We again pulled the family together. The sons listened carefully, amidst the chorus of tears, and decided that she should take the risk. I made sure that this was also her choice, and she seemed surprisingly comfortable with it. "If the Lord wants me to join my husband, then I will have to go." Once she made up her mind, there was no turning back. She went through the surgery without complications. The tumor turned out to be an isolated plasmacytoma, a cancer that was fully curable once removed. Mrs. Martinez had again cheated death, and she was thrilled to be alive. She felt that God and her doctors were in partnership, watching over her to ensure her safety. Although she wanted repeated assurances over the next year that the residual pain in her scar did not represent a return of her cancer, she resumed her normal life of socializing with her friends and family.

The next major medical event in Mrs. Martinez's life was the loss of one of her best friends to cancer. Her friend died at home, supported by her family and the hospice workers, but in her last weeks she was delirious, confined to bed, yelling out much of the time. Mrs. Martinez would not want that end for herself. I assured her that I would do my best to relieve any potential suffering should she need that kind of help in the future. I also suggested that, given her family's ardent wish that she live forever, she complete an advance directive. I recommended that she put down her wishes in the form of a living will, and that she name a family member to act on her behalf in the form of a health care proxy.[1] Not surprisingly, Mrs. Martinez wanted her oldest son to be her proxy. At my recommendation, we had a joint meeting with her son. I wanted to avert a clash of cultures by achieving a joint understanding that the

1. Samples of these documents are included in the Appendix.

son's job, if Mrs. Martinez lost the ability to speak for herself, was to represent *her* wishes, and not his own or the family's wishes, as best he could. In order to do so, he would have to acquire a deeper understanding of his mother's future wishes, fears, and values. Mrs. Martinez's son was very receptive to the inquiry. He was feeling the burden of potentially having to make such decisions in a vacuum and be subject to the second guessing of his siblings. The three of us achieved a mutual understanding and completed both documents. At the end of the meeting Mrs. Martinez again proclaimed her love for me and gave me a hug and a kiss as her son laughed appreciatively.

Two years later Mrs. Martinez had her most frightening encounter with cancer to date. Her youngest son, who had also been a heavy smoker and drinker, developed oral cancer. Mrs. Martinez wept throughout her next visit. How could God have done this? How could a mother outlive her son? She was again feeling anxious and was unable to sleep. "This has me really nervous! I don't know if I can handle this." Her faith in God was being tested, and she felt like giving up. We talked about the prognosis of her son's illness; since it had been caught early, there was a good chance that it could be cured. We also agreed to meet more regularly until her son's condition was better understood.

Two months later Mrs. Martinez was admitted to the hospital with fever and abdominal pain. Her liver was enlarged, and there were multiple cystic lesions. The lesions appeared to have been caused by liver abscesses, but cancer was also possible. We arranged for a liver biopsy using a thin needle that could be directly guided into one of the cysts. The biopsy showed a very aggressive form of primary liver cancer. The diagnosis was subsequently supported by a very high level of *alpha fetal protein*, a tumor marker in the blood.

From a medical perspective, it all made sense. These tumors are common in patients with cirrhosis of the liver, which Mrs. Martinez had had for over twenty years. Perhaps it was manifesting itself now because her immune defenses were being suppressed as she grieved over her son's illness. Yet at an irrational level it didn't add up. We had been through so many scrapes together that we both subconsciously believed that our relationship would somehow guarantee Mrs. Martinez safe passage.

What should I tell her, and how? The medical facts were not promising. Treatment for this cancer is generally ineffective. Surgical removal is sometimes possible, though in Mrs. Martinez's case, because of the multiple sites and the already damaged liver, it was out of the question. Palliative chemotherapy is often offered, but it remains largely ineffective. There were no cures; at best, we could temporarily suppress the disease. In our private meetings before the procedure, Mrs. Martinez had said that she wanted to know the results even if it was cancer. Her family, however, felt that she should not be told. "It would kill her to know if it is cancer." I told them I would have to tell her the truth if she asked. I also thought that it would be better if she knew, since such secrets are virtually impossible to keep. Mrs. Martinez said she would like to have her oldest son and her pastor present when we talked about the results. I was not at all sure what to expect from our exchange. I would go slowly, feeling my way.

We sat down together. Mrs. Martinez knew from my appearance that the news was not good.

"It's cancer, isn't it?" she asked in a matter-of-fact tone.

"Are you sure you want to know?" I asked.

"Yes."

"It is cancer," I told her, confirming what she already knew.

"How bad is it?" she wondered aloud.

"It is not one for which there is easy treatment." I told her the truth as gently as I knew how.

"I thought so."

Mrs. Martinez asked for and got the information she needed in small, digestible pieces. Although her eyes glistened, she remained fully composed. Her main concern was how her family would absorb the news. Her pastor asked for some clarification about some of the medical issues and then restated them in Spanish to be sure that Mrs. Martinez understood. We talked about experimental chemotherapy and about comfort-oriented care. Mrs. Martinez asked what I recom-

mended. I suggested that she discuss her situation with our medical oncologists so that she would understand all the available options but ven-
tured that comfort care would probably be her best choice. She agreed
to see the oncologists, but she had already decided that she wanted no
invasive treatment. She wanted to put herself in God's hands, hoping
for a miracle but accepting what came. That sounded like a sane approach to me, one that would avoid unnecessary suffering. We parted
with our ritual hug, committed to facing the future together.

My next challenge was to face her family, waiting in the next room.
Upon hearing that it was cancer, they immediately fell apart, scream-
ing at God and begging me not to tell them this. "I can't live without
her!" As the crying, pleading, and lamenting dissipated, the Martinez
family again began to work its magic. Those who were quiet were
hugged and made part of the process. Those in the greatest outward
pain were comforted by the strongest. Although this was overwhelming news, they gradually came to grips with it. As they got past their
own pain, they began to wonder how Mrs. Martinez had taken the
news. They agreed to stay strong and collectively help care for her. Mrs.
Martinez wanted to remain in her own apartment as long as possible.
Plans were made to come up with a schedule of visits by all family
members, young and old. They got up the courage to face Mrs. Martinez, which they did two at a time until all the family members had
paid their respects. Her position as matriarch of the extended family
was never clearer. Taking guidance from Mrs. Martinez's acceptance
of her fate, many in the family found the courage to make the final
journey with her. Since Mrs. Martinez would be living alone at first,
we postponed the formal referral to hospice. She did not want to be
part of a formal program. For now she would be supported by her family and community health nurses.

Mrs. Martinez visited the office with her son two weeks later. She
was losing weight, and the family was pressuring her to eat more. We
had a long talk about the goals of her treatment and about the importance of focusing our energy entirely on enhancing the quality of her
life. This could best be done by offering her small amounts of her fa-

vorite foods and not overemphasizing the number of calories or exact content. Mrs. Martinez was not interested in protein supplements, but she did have a sweet tooth, which I encouraged them to indulge.

Two weeks later, having become very jaundiced, Mrs. Martinez became too weak to walk independently. She was briefly hospitalized, and at a family meeting we explored her options. No one wanted her to go to a nursing home, but most family members were hesitant to take her into their own homes. Most of the adults were employed, and the few who were not working had significant problems with alcohol and anxiety. We eventually got beyond the logistics of caring for Mrs. Martinez and focused on their fears. None of them had been around a dying person, and they were at a loss about what to expect or do. The presence of a formal hospice program to assist and guide them at home now became very important. After considerable negotiation and soul searching, the second-oldest son and his wife decided to take Mrs. Martinez to their home. A hospital bed was set up in their daughter's bedroom on the first floor, and the entire family promised to help out. The daughter-in-law took a leave of absence from work to become the primary caregiver, and home visits from hospice workers were scheduled. Mrs. Martinez would now be in God's hands.

Mrs. Martinez's initial time on hospice included daily visits from family and friends. There was little explicit talk about death and dying. Instead, old family stories were told, including those about the many storms they had weathered together. Mrs. Martinez had private meetings with each of her children and grandchildren, during which she imparted words of her wisdom to them. After six weeks I received a telephone call telling me that Mrs. Martinez's pain was worsening and the family wanted to bring her to the hospital. The offer of a home visit was gratefully accepted. When I arrived, I found an ideal hospice scene. Mrs. Martinez's bedroom was on the first floor right off the living room, in the center of the daily activity. Family pictures were all around her, and there were chairs for her frequent visitors. She was neatly dressed in a sleeping gown, and she had small glasses of various liquids on a table next to her bed. She was experiencing more pain in her liver, but her pain medicines could easily be increased. Mrs. Martinez complained primarily of feeling weak and tired, but otherwise her symptom control was very good. She wanted to return to her own apartment, yet she was unable even to get out of bed independently. When I asked her what was wrong, she admitted that the current arrangement just wasn't working out.

I left her bedroom to talk privately with the family. The majority of Mrs. Martinez's care had fallen upon one daughter-in-law, and she was exhausted. She was going to lose her job if she did not return the next week. Their teenage daughter, who had given up her room for her grandmother, was feeling displaced and fearful about having someone die in her room. In addition, the remaining family members had not lived up to their promise to share the responsibilities of Mrs. Martinez's care. We explored the options, including hospitalization, which nobody really wanted. Our best choice was to allow Mrs. Martinez to return to her own apartment. Her oldest son agreed to stay with her, providing primary care and coordinating the visits of other family members. Since he was now the dominant family decision maker, having him oversee the visit routine seemed ideal. Although he was inexperienced in the realities of hands-on care, he was genuinely willing to try if that was what his mother wanted. When the idea was presented to Mrs. Martinez, she wept in gratitude. Her dream was to spend her last days in her own home of almost fifty years.

The move home worked out surprisingly well. Most family members participated in the scheduled visits. The oldest son carried the burden but also received the rewards of being the primary caregiver. It was an exhausting task, sometimes exasperating, other times exhilarating. The opportunity to connect with and care for his mother would never be forgotten. Gradually, as Mrs. Martinez became harder to arouse, I was asked to pay another home visit. Upon arriving, I was greeted by the son, who appeared tired and tearful. "I think the end is near. She has stopped eating and drinking. What should I do?" I reassured him that continuing to "be with" his mother for her last days was most important. Stopping eating and drinking was a natural end to the life cycle and was not associated with any added suffering. I suggested that this phase of the dying process was usually harder on the family than on the patient. We would continue her opioids to avoid any chance of her being in pain. There was no need to hospitalize her for intravenous fluids. The best thing we could do was to continue to support her at home and allow her to die as gently as possible. I emphasized that she was very lucky to have a son and family who were willing to come through for her at the end.

I then went in to see Mrs. Martinez. She was a shadow of her former self. Smaller, thinner, more wrinkled, and bright yellow. She appeared to be sleeping, so I simply held her hand. Death would come soon, and she appeared to be at peace. It had been a long adventure, but we had done a good job. She then opened her eyes, looked straight at me, and smiled. She still had a twinkle in her eye and a charming attractiveness in her smile. She gazed at me silently for a few minutes. "Do you still love me?" she asked. "Of course, I do." I responded. I then gave her a final kiss and hug. She closed her eyes, smiling faintly, and went back to sleep.

She died quietly two days later, her family at her bedside.

Commentary

1. *From her deathbed, Mrs. Martinez asked if I still loved her.* Although I don't believe it is possible or desirable to love all my patients, this term of affection is clearly accurate for some, and Mrs. Martinez was one of those. *Love* in this context describes a special friendship, characterized by deep affinity, that can develop over time between doctor and patient. This bond of personal commitment and connection supplements the more professional requirements of the doctor-patient relationship, such as integrity, confidentiality, informed consent, and medical competence. The doctor comes to know the patient as a friend as well as a patient, and what happens to him or her takes on an emotional and existential complexity that enriches the practice of medicine. This more intimate

approach to patient care is a powerful antidote to the remoteness of excessive professionalism.

Physicians who choose to utilize this more personal approach to patient care need to be aware of the risks of overinvolvement. They must guard against losing the objectivity they need if they are to be competent medical guides for their patients. The pain of losing too many "good friends" may become draining rather than enriching. Not wishing to burden their "friend" with another complaint, patients may avoid conflict to protect the relationship. Conversely, doctors may become tempted to violate clear professional prohibitions against sexual involvement with patients for whom they feel a romantic attraction. Countertransference is an issue not only in psychiatric relationships; it is present in medical relationships as well. Doctors need to be able to confidentially discuss and explore their closest doctor-patient relationships with trusted colleagues so that appropriate professional boundaries are maintained. Once a middle ground can be found between excessive professional detachment and overinvolvement, doctors may discover that their practice has become more meaningful and enriching.

A wider range of end-of-life decisions can be entertained if there is a trust and interpersonal connection between doctor and patient. Aggressive medical treatment is sometimes continued too long because it seems safer and easier in the short term than having the difficult discussions about the limitations of medical therapy and the inevitability of death. Moving from potentially life-sustaining therapy to a comfort-oriented approach requires a leap of faith that one is not giving up too soon. It also requires a clear vision of what one is choosing instead of traditional treatment. Mrs. Martinez and her family knew clearly that I had her best interests at heart and would not abandon them under any circumstances. Choosing hospice instead of chemotherapy or surgery was a stretch for several family members, for they had never experienced a peaceful, accepting approach to death. They had to overcome both their wish that medical care would be more powerful and their fear that death would inevitably be harsh and humiliating. Had we not had the twelve years of shared experience, this leap of faith might not have been possible.

On her deathbed Mrs. Martinez may also have been asking if she was still *loveable*. Many dying patients feel that their various deformities and infirmities have made them grotesque, disgusting, or appalling. Some members of Mrs. Martinez's family feared that cancer could be transmitted by casual contact, which made them reluctant to touch or hug her. Sometimes health care providers are the only ones who provide a human touch for a dying patient. Many home health aides and nurses are the central providers of this vital, healing, physical contact. Although Mrs. Martinez's body was disintegrating, her personhood continued to grow stronger and more complete as death approached. Because we had taught them to be less afraid of her physical deterioration, the members of her family were able to stay close and learn from her throughout the dying process. She gave her children words of wisdom to help them in their individual life journeys. Her grandchildren were able to climb up on the bed and learn that death was not necessarily something to fear. She gave me another reminder of what sustains me in the path that I have chosen.

2. *Communication barriers can impede mutual decision making between patients and their doctors.* Many obstacles were present in my initial encounters with Mrs. Martinez. Not only were our cultural and socioeconomic backgrounds different, but we appeared not even to speak the same language. Helping patients to make informed decisions is difficult enough when one is working in the world of uncertain medical odds and outcomes. Such decisions are confounded when they include a subtext of having to face one's own mortality and medicine's inherent limitations. These conversations are exponentially complicated by the addition of a translator, who potentially brings his or her own biases to each subject and who may have a preexisting, complex relationship with the patient. Our initial translator was Mrs. Martinez's daughter, who had a very close but ambivalent relationship with her mother. Their interpersonal dynamics added to our already formidable list of barriers. Later, as Mrs. Martinez faced the decision about hos-

pice versus experimental therapy, her pastor served as a more skilled, unbiased translator. She could confirm and explore in Spanish what I hoped had been communicated in English, ensuring more complete mutual understanding.

In overcoming barriers, there is no substitute for shared experience. The death of Mrs. Martinez's husband on the operating table could have irrevocably threatened our slowly emerging relationship. Instead, it solidified our commitment to one another, demonstrating that we would stick together in the face of adversity. My personal challenge at that time was to accept the overwhelming emotional response by the family without taking it personally and then to respond to Mrs. Martinez's fears about being newly widowed and alone. The family's challenge was to believe that I had not led them astray by guiding Mr. Martinez toward the surgery that resulted in his death. Their style of grieving initially made me very uncomfortable. By caring and responding as best I could, given my own cultural and experiential limitations, I managed to earn their trust. This enabled me to guide them through the uncertain medical terrain as Mrs. Martinez's future unfolded.

3. *The Martinez family did not want their mother to know she had cancer.* "It would kill her to know! She could not handle it!" It would have been easy to accede to this request. They are the experts concerning how such information is handled in their family and culture. Yet Western medical ethics teaches that patients have a right to be fully informed so that they can make their own decisions. Fortunately, I knew Mrs. Martinez well enough to challenge their assumption, and I assured them I would tell her only what she wanted to know. In this particular situation there were serious questions about who was being protected—the family or the patient. Besides, if we tried to keep her diagnosis a secret from her, Mrs. Martinez would sense that something was drastically wrong. As her symptoms increased, she would probably guess the diagnosis anyway and would then be put in the position of isolating herself further to protect the family secret.

When I asked Mrs. Martinez if she wanted to discuss the results of the biopsy, her immediate response was "It's cancer, isn't it?" Not only did she know,but she was very clear about what approach she wanted once she understood the inherent limitations of aggressive medical treatment. Although she ardently hoped for a miracle, her miracle would come from God, not from modern medicine. She was calm and accepting. Her main concern was how her children who had emotional problems would handle it. Given her lifelong fear of cancer, her past problems with anxiety, and her family's dire predictions, Mrs. Martinez's outward equanimity was unexpected. Yet, allowing her the opportunity to face the truth about her condition enabled her to make an informed decision that defined the landmarks of the last phase of her life.

4. *Hospice is the standard of care when patients choose to forgo aggressive medical care.* Hospice offers a radically different approach to the last phase in one's life that emphasizes the quality over the quantity of the time that remains. Some patients (like Cynthia) make an informed choice for aggressive treatment even when the odds of success are very small. But others may choose it because they don't want to disappoint their doctors or because they worry that they will be abandoned by the medical system if they give up on treatment. Hospice should be a powerful antidote to the fear of abandonment, for a wide range of resources can be brought to bear to support the terminally ill patient and his or her family.

"Comfort care" is the general philosophy that underlies hospice and palliative care. Symptoms such as pain, shortness of breath, and nausea are aggressively treated in this approach. All treatments and interventions that do not directly contribute to the patient's quality of life are discontinued. Once symptoms are controlled, comfort care emphasizes human contact and support, helping each person achieve a meaningful closure to life according to his or her own values and wishes. If the patient has a prognosis of six months or less and there is a primary caregiver at home, the patient may be referred to a formal hospice program. Then the resources of a multidisciplinary team, including physicians, nurses, home health aides, social workers, clergy, and volunteers, can be brought to bear. The support and expertise of such teams can be invaluable. Comfort care, however, is a philosophy of care that can be applied in any setting or program.

The quality of a patient's last months often is determined by whether an aggressive approach or a comfort-oriented approach is chosen. Instead of hospitalizations, blood tests, chemotherapy, and other invasive treatments that were unlikely to help, Mrs. Martinez received around-the-clock pain medicine and frequent visits from family and friends. The opportunity to put her life in perspective was enhanced by the support of experienced hospice professionals. She eventually accepted that it was her time to die and that she would soon be joining her husband. Her family, so devastated by the initial diagnosis, was able to spend time with their mother and grandmother, knowing that their time together was limited and therefore precious. The family learned that death need not always be harsh but can sometimes be enriching and uplifting. The son who had recently been diagnosed with oral cancer now had a wider range of experience to bring to his own uncertain future.

References

Empathy and Connection

American Board of Internal Medicine, Subcommittee on Evaluation of Humanistic Qualities in the Internist. Evaluation of humanistic qualities in the internist. *Annals of Internal Medicine* 99 (1983): 720–24.

Bellet, P. S., and M. J. Maloney. The importance of empathy as an interviewing skill in medicine. *Journal of the American Medical Association* 266 (1991): 1831–32.

Benjamin, W. W. Healing by the fundamentals. *New England Journal of Medicine* 311 (1984): 595–97.

Branch, W. T., and A. L. Suchman. Meaningful experiences in medicine. *American Journal of Medicine* 88 (1990): 56–59.

Matthews, D. A., A. L. Suchman, and W. T. Branch. Making "connexions": Enhancing the therapeutic potential of patient-clinician relationships. *Annals of Internal Medicine* 118 (1993): 973–77.

Zinn, W. The empathic physician. *Archives of Internal Medicine* 153 (1993): 306–12.

Barriers

Barsky, A. J. Hidden reasons some patients visit doctors. *Annals of Internal Medicine* 94 (1981): 492–98.

Kraut, A. M. Healers and strangers: Immigrant attitudes toward the physician in America—a relationship in historical perspective. *Journal of the American Medical Association* 263 (1990): 1807–11.

Lazare, A. Shame and humiliation in the medical encounter. *Archives of Internal Medicine* 147 (1987): 1653–58.

Quill, T. E. Recognizing and adjusting to barriers in doctor-patient communication. *Annals of Internal Medicine* 111 (1989): 51–57.

Truth-Telling

Kleinman, A. The cultural meanings and social uses of illness: A role for medical anthropology and clinically oriented social science in the development of primary care theory and research. *Journal of Family Practice* 16 (1983): 539–45.

————. *Patients and Healers in the Context of Culture: An Exploration of the Borderland between Anthropology, Medicine, and Psychiatry.* Berkeley: University of California Press, 1980.

Kraut, A. M. Healers and strangers: Immigrant attitudes toward the physician in America—a relationship in historical perspective. *Journal of the American Medical Association* 263 (1990): 1807–11.

Pellegrino, E. D. Is truth telling to the patient a cultural artifact? *Journal of the American Medical Association* 268 (1992): 1734–35.

Surbone, A. Truth telling to the patient. *Journal of the American Medical Association* 268 (1992): 1661–62.

Tong, K. L. The Chinese palliative patient and family in North America: A cultural perspective. *Journal of Palliative Care* 10 (1994): 26–28.

Hospice Is the Standard of Care for the Dying

Broadfield, L. Evaluation of palliative care: Current status and future directions. *Journal of Palliative Care* 4 (1988): 21–28.

Christakis, N. A. Timing of referral of terminally ill patients to an outpatient hospice. *Journal of General Internal Medicine* 9 (1994): 314–20.

Cohen, S. R., and B. M. Mount. Quality of life in terminal illness: Defining and measuring subjective well-being in the dying. *Journal of Palliative Care* 8 (1992): 40–45.

Council on Scientific Affairs, American Medical Association. Good care of the dying patient. *Journal of the American Medical Association* 275 (1996): 474–78.

Kane, R. L., L. Bernstein, J. Wales, and R. Rothenberg. Hospice effectiveness in controlling pain. *Journal of the American Medical Association* 253 (1985): 2683–86.

Miller, F. G., T. E. Quill, H. Brody, J. C. Fletcher, L. O. Gostin, and D. E. Meier. Regulating physician-assisted death. *New England Journal of Medicine* 331 (1994): 119–23.

Morris, J. N., V. Mor, R. J. Goldberg, S. Sherwood, D. S. Greer, and J. Hiris. The effect of treatment setting and patient characteristics on pain in terminal cancer patients: A report from the National Hospice Study. *Journal of Chronic Diseases* 39 (1986): 27–35.

Quill, T. E., C. K. Cassel, and D. E. Meier. Care of the hopelessly ill: Proposed criteria for physician-assisted suicide. *New England Journal of Medicine* 327 (1992): 1380–84.

Rhymes, J. Hospice care in America. *Journal of the American Medical Association* 264 (1990): 369–72.

Seale, C. F. What happens in hospices: A review of research evidence. *Social Science and Medicine* 28 (1989): 551–59.

Chapter 4

It Took a Lickin' and Kept on Tickin'

QUESTIONS ABOUT SUICIDE have always plagued and intrigued
philosophers, ethicists, lawyers, and clinicians. Is the wish for death
inevitably a sign of mental illness, or can it be rational under some adverse circumstances? Is it suicide when a terminally ill patient chooses
to take his or her life in the face of intolerable, untreatable suffering? To
protect the sanctity of life, should we resist any direct easing of death
no matter how devastating the patient's circumstances? If we do help
patients who wish to die, how do we proceed and still maintain important ethical, professional, and legal boundaries?

Several clinicians were struggling with these questions in their efforts to respond to Mr. Williams' wish to die. His wish was complicated
because he had an implantable cardiac defibrillator, a wonder of advanced medical technology that electrically restarted his heart each
time it developed a life-threatening arrhythmia.[1] In Mr. Williams' eyes
the issue was simple and personal. He wanted his defibrillator turned
off so that he could die in peace, with what little dignity he still had. His
life had become a living hell. With so many disabilities, symptoms, and
limitations, he was unable to participate meaningfully in daily life. There
were no realistic prospects of improvement or recovery.

For his cardiologists the questions were mainly legal and ethical.
Discontinuing his defibrillator would help Mr. Williams achieve a
wished-for death. If they deactivated the device, wouldn't they be as-

---

1. A brief version of this case was published in a cardiology journal along with a discussion of the clinical, ethical, and legal issues (see T. E. Quill, S. S. Barold, and B. Sussman, Discontinuing an implantable cardioverter-defibrillator as a life-sustaining treatment,
American Journal of Cardiology 74 [1994]: 205–7).

sisting him in suicide and therefore be legally vulnerable and morally suspect? For his psychiatrist the dilemmas were confounded by clinical questions about his mental competence. Can it ever be rational to want to die, or is it by definition a sign of mental illness? Many severely ill patients are discouraged, if not clinically depressed. Should such sadness always disqualify them from making serious life-and-death decisions about their medical care? If they are to be excluded from these determinations, then who should make them? Unfortunately, there were more questions than answers, and Mr. Williams' requests were therefore avoided and minimized.

I first saw Mr. Williams as an ethics consultant because of my long-standing interest in end-of-life decision making. Ordinarily, I do not formally consult with patients who wish to die, because I do not want to become known as a specialist in these matters. However, I agreed to see Mr. Williams after hearing an overview of his situation from his main cardiologist, who was willing to turn off the defibrillator if I determined that doing so was ethically, legally, and clinically appropriate.

I met with Mr. Williams and his wife only once. In anticipation of his appointment, I reviewed the medical reports of his hospitalizations and office visits. I also read assessments by two psychiatrists attesting to Mr. Williams' mental competence. It was tempting to resolve this question based on the fundamental ethical premise that competent patients have the right to refuse unwanted therapy. Yet, the only way to understand this man's clinical and existential situation well enough to help with a decision of this magnitude was to hear him tell his story. The details of a person's history provide a context that gives life and meaning to our ethical principles.

Mr. Williams' physical appearance was striking. A large man, he was squeezed into a wheelchair, where he now spent most of his life. His body was swollen from the side effects of corticosteroid medication. His skin, which would begin to bleed at the slightest touch, was covered with large reddish brown patches (ecchymoses). He labored to breathe, and the least exertion, even talking, left him exhausted. An oxygen tank connected to his nose by a long green tube was always with him. He lived with chronic back pain from the many collapsed vertebrae in his spine. Any movement, even shifting in his chair, would produce shocks of pain that extended down his legs. The basic task of having a bowel movement, which he performed in a bedpan placed on his wheelchair, was overwhelming.

In spite of his many disabilities, Mr. Williams established good eye contact and engaged readily in our conversation. He was not pleased to have to see another doctor, but he hoped this consultation would be the last hurdle in his struggle to be allowed to die.

Mr. Williams had always been an active man. A toolmaker by profession, he was an avid hunter and fisherman. His father had had a heart attack at a relatively young age, but Mr. Williams never worried much about such matters. He smoked heavily and ate whatever he wanted. Workdays were long, and he would usually stop for a few beers with his co-workers on his way home. Married in his early twenties, he had helped his wife raise their three children, two of whom had gone to college. Periodically he had felt trapped by his job and family responsibilities, but the anticipation of retirement had always sustained him. The couple's children had finally become financially independent just before Mr. Williams became sick for the first time.

Mr. Williams' first heart attack occurred in 1975, when he was fifty. It came as a complete shock to him. He had never even contemplated becoming seriously ill, much less facing his own mortality. Thirty percent of his heart was damaged, and his life was further threatened by irregularities in his heartbeat. As was the custom at that time, he was immobilized in the coronary care unit for five days, staying in the hospital for a total of two weeks. The passivity required in such a setting undermined how he defined himself. Deprived of his usual outlets and distractions, he became very discouraged. Mr. Williams was told that he should not smoke, drink alcohol, or eat foods that contained cholesterol. When he learned that his physical activity would also be limited for several months, he became clinically depressed. He had been asked to give up so many things that were important to him. What, if anything, would take their place? Mr. Williams did not usually discuss his feelings and concerns. Seeing no way out, he began to feel so hopeless and withdrawn that he accepted a brief psychiatric hospitalization.

After he returned home, Mr. Williams began to work with a psychiatrist who seemed to understand what he was facing. He learned to give voice to some of his inner experience and accepted the challenge of finding a way through his recovery. Mr. Williams was started on an antidepressant medication, which initially helped him to sleep better and later was associated with a considerable improvement in his mood. After four months he returned to work part-time. Instead of feeling like his old robust self, however, he found himself easily fatigued and distracted. Eventually he was able to work full-time, but work no longer was easy for him. He felt so exhausted that his weekends were spent trying to recuperate so that he could face the next week.

Mr. Williams consulted his cardiologist regularly during this period. Although he did not have another documented heart attack, his heart function deteriorated inexplicably. His doctors performed a cardiac catheterization to see if he could be helped by open-heart surgery. Unfortunately, the blocked arteries they found in his heart could not be opened mechanically or bypassed. He simultaneously developed life-threatening arrhythmias, erratic, ineffective series of heartbeats associated with a severe drop in blood pressure, which often left him feeling lightheaded and exhausted. Multiple medications were tried to stabilize his heart rhythm, but most had side effects and none were effective. By 1978 Mr. Williams was no longer able to work as a toolmaker. He had no skills that translated easily to more sedentary work. Besides, his severe medical problems made him a "poor candidate for job retraining." He requested and received Social Security disability.

Mr. Williams adjusted surprisingly well to premature retirement and his reduced physical abilities. He and his wife took several trips, and he developed an interest in bird-watching, a hobby he could pursue even when his physical activity needed to be severely restricted. Life was not what he had hoped it would be, but he found enough meaning and enjoyment to carry on. He restricted his intake of sodium and fats and almost completely gave up cigarettes (although he would occasionally sneak one or two to affirm his independence). "I have to have at least one small vice since I have given up everything else," he explained.

Mr. Williams' heart disease remained relatively stable for the next few years, but several new problems further compromised his already diminished quality of life. He developed both asthma and emphysema, which initially could be controlled with inhalers but eventually required both systemic corticosteroids and continuous oxygen. The corticosteroids aggravated his tendency to gain weight, and he ballooned larger than ever. The medicine also contributed to his developing osteoporosis, a thinning of the bones that made them vulnerable to fracture. He already had intermittent back pain from degenerative arthritis of the lower spine, but now the bones in his back would periodically collapse, escalating the degree of his pain from tolerable to overwhelming. The severe pain of each compression fracture would last about six weeks. During these intense periods he was unable to distract himself by watching television, much less by bird-watching or talking with family and friends.

Mr. Williams somehow managed to adjust to the narrowing confines of his life. He and his wife grew very close, sharing their thoughts and feelings as never before. Although he would at times be irritable, they learned how to work around each other during the bad times and to find enjoyment together when he was feeling relatively well. Life was far from what they had had in mind for retirement but better than his not being alive at all.

In 1989 Mr. Williams developed ventricular tachycardia, a severe cardiac arrhythmia that would cause him to lose consciousness without warning. He was admitted to the hospital to try to suppress these erratic heartbeats with medication. A series of antiarrhythmic drugs, both traditional and experimental, were unsuccessful. His life was saved several times when the cardiologists electrically shocked his fibrillating heart back into a regular heart rhythm.

Mr. Williams was told that the only way to prevent repeated fainting spells, and probably his eventual death, was to insert a mechanical device that could detect arrhythmias, electrically disrupt them, and then allow a more normal heart rhythm to resume. Without this device, sudden death would likely occur once he left the constant monitoring of the hospital. With the machine he would live longer, for it would automatically restart his heart as the cardiologists had done. The procedure was not without risk, however, because it required major surgery to implant a mechanical device into his abdomen and then attach it with wires directly to his heart. (More recently developed devices are considerably smaller and safer to insert.) Given Mr. Williams' frail heart and his emphysema, he might not survive the surgery. But it was the only thing left to offer. His cardiologist was enthusiastic and did not see any reasonable alternatives.

Mr. Williams consented to the surgery and survived it with surprising ease. Everyone was pleased with the outcome. The cardiologist saw the implanted defibrillator as another example of the seemingly unlimited potential of advanced cardiac technology. The Williams family, who had grown to know their father and husband in a more complex and personal way over the past ten years of illness, saw the device as a way to keep him alive for an added period of time. Even Mr. Williams was initially pleased. For once, at least, things had gone more easily than anticipated.

For the next two years Mr. Williams' condition remained relatively stable. He avoided hospitalization and suffered no major deterioration. He could go shopping with his wife, although he now needed a wheelchair whenever he moved more than a few feet. Their three children and their families would come from out of town for short stays. Unfortunately, their visits were often more exhausting than enjoyable because of Mr. Williams' extreme physical limitations and medical care needs. For the most part, Mr. Williams and his wife were on their own, with the exception of the community health nurses and home health aides. The nurses monitored his clinical condition and the complex regimen of medications and inhalers, now totaling over forty doses each day. The home health aides had to assist him with all of his personal care, from dressing to bathing. The members of the health care team became his friends as well as caregivers, and he looked forward to the distraction and companionship their daily visits provided. Mrs. Williams used their visits as an opportunity to get a breath of fresh air, temporarily escaping the round-the-clock job into which her husband's care had evolved. Although Mr. Williams' medical needs were at times relentless, his wife was not resentful, seeing them simply as an extension of her role as a mother and wife. She found great meaning in his care and in their relationship. In her rare private moments she wondered how she would cope when he finally died.

Showers were a major undertaking for Mr. Williams and his caregivers. He had to get his large body, and all his medical paraphernalia, into the shower, where a seat was set up. Once he was seated, the water could be run over him and, assisted by a home health aide, he would painstakingly wash himself. Ordinarily a very private, modest person, he amazed both himself and his wife by adjusting to being physically cared for by strangers.

The implantable defibrillator went off only twice during the first year and three times in the second. Each episode was both physically and psychologically disturbing. Suddenly, out of the blue, Mr. Williams would feel very lightheaded. He then got a powerful electrical shock, which left him disoriented for several hours. One day, seated in the shower, he felt he was about to faint. His heart was beating erratically; it would only be a moment before the defibrillator would go off. Having had considerable experience with electricity, he knew that having his feet in water would ground the electrical charge. But there was nothing he could do! He experienced a moment of terror and then the most severe jolt he had ever had! He lost consciousness and fell off the chair onto the floor of the tub. The home health aide ran to his side. His pulse was now normal, but he was unresponsive. She then tried to get this mountain of a man out of the tub to a safer place.

Mr. Williams gradually regained consciousness. He was sprawled out on the bathroom floor, naked and bleeding. The excruciating pain in his back meant that he had additional compression fractures. He felt ashamed and humiliated. Thoughts and questions he had been suppressing suddenly emerged with startling clarity. "What is the point?"

"How can I possibly go on living this way?" "This really isn't living!" "Death must be better than this!"

Over the next six months the unthinkable began to grow. Mr. Williams' chronic back pain left him so incapacitated that he left the house only for doctor's appointments. Pain medicine for arthritis would irritate his stomach, and stronger pain relievers would cloud his consciousness and make him constipated. Every intervention designed to help him feel better had unintended side effects, complicating his life and taking away what little quality remained. He talked to his psychiatrist about his growing discouragement and the loss of meaning in his life. He was diagnosed with a reactive depression and again started on antidepressant medication. The medicine helped a little, but it couldn't make up for how irrevocably diminished his life had become. Even lying down in bed became an ordeal, so he began sleeping sitting up in his wheelchair. Although he did not really want to die, he did not want to live under these circumstances.

Meanwhile, every month or two Mr. Williams would get dizzy, nearly fainting, and his implanted defibrillator would go off, once again saving his life. As he emerged from the confusion that this ritual induced, he became angry and afraid. "There is no way I can die with this thing restarting my heart each time it tries to stop. This could go on forever." He thought of suicide but ruled it out for religious reasons. Mr. Williams was a devout Catholic, and suicide was a mortal sin, to be avoided even in the face of intolerable agony. He then realized that the only way he could die "naturally" would be to have this device taken out or turned off. Once the idea occurred to him, it became an obsession. His wife initially countered that she couldn't bear to lose him, and she reassured him that his ongoing care needs had become a meaningful part of her life. But she gradually began to listen empathically to his persistent plea. He was a shadow of his former self, deprived of everything that had meaning except her love and caring. And there was no end in sight because of this damn defibrillator! While it was not what she wanted, Mrs. Williams eventually decided that she would support his right to choose.

How could Mr. Williams bring this up with his cardiologists? These doctors had worked hard to keep him alive and were enthusiastic about the success of their experimental device. Would they think he was crazy or just ungrateful? Might they declare him suicidal and commit him to a mental institution? Despite the risk that his request might be misinterpreted, Mr. Williams eventually broached the subject with his cardiologist. "My life has gotten so bad that I want to die, and I need your help by turning off my defibrillator." His first foray was dismissed out of hand. "You are simply going through a bad patch. Let's see what happens over the next several months." When his request became more persistent, the cardiologists tried a different tact. "We should increase your antidepressant medication. You should see your psychiatrist more often." When the requests continued, the doctors resorted to their (mis)perception of the law. "It is illegal to help patients to commit suicide. We wish we could help you, but we can't. Our hands are tied. Once these things are started, there is no way to stop them."

At this juncture Mr. Williams gave up. He wanted to die but felt forced to have his life prolonged by advanced medical technology. The hope that the cardiologists might help him to die peacefully by deactivating the defibrillator had sustained him for the last several months. He now fell into a much deeper depression. He was trapped in a dark world with no windows and no doors. Meaning and joy had disappeared, and there was no way out. And it could only get worse. All of his medical problems were progressive: cardiomyopathy, emphysema, osteoporosis and the associated back pain. He could not even die a natural death because his ailing heart would automatically be restarted by his implanted defibrillator.

Deprived of any other option, Mr. Williams became preoccupied with suicide. In his weakened condition, religious prohibition began to fade and he began to search for methods. He had guns but no ammunition. Asking for ammunition would clearly give him away. Besides, the violence of such a death would leave an irrevocable mark on his wife and family, whom he was determined not to harm. He had some diazepam (Valium), which he thought would be lethal in overdose. At his wit's end, Mr. Williams took twenty tablets all at once. Several hours later, when not much had happened, he took two hundred more. When he became sleepier, his wife discovered what had happened and called an ambulance. In the emergency department a tube was forced into Mr. Williams' stomach to pump out the undigested medication. He was also given a cathartic to remove any remaining unabsorbed pills, as well as an antidote to the diazepam. He had once again been saved by medical intervention. Now the medical challenge was to help him find the will to live.

His psychiatrist listened to his painful story. Mr. Williams was now clinically depressed, and death dominated his thoughts. Yet he also had an accurate grasp of his medical condition and prognosis. He said that he had felt "empty" for several years but had nevertheless managed to cope until six months earlier, when his doctors had refused his request to have his defibrillator discontinued. At that point he had lost all hope of finding a way through the nightmare his life had become. Although Mr. Williams had the support of his family and no financial worries, his health was so irreversibly compromised that it seemed impossible to go on living. He openly admitted being disappointed that the overdose had not worked but promised not to attempt it again and to give a new medication for depression a chance. Mr. Williams also agreed to resume more intensive psychotherapy to further explore his predicament. As part of their therapeutic agreement, his psychiatrist promised to support his wish to have his defibrillator discontinued if it persisted even after his depression was better treated. This promise, more than anything else, gave Mr. Williams a glimmer of hope.

Mr. Williams fully complied with the recommended treatment program. Several of the newer serotonin-uptake-inhibitor antidepressants were prescribed; he experienced some improvement in his mood and no discernible side effects. In spite of the physical ordeal of getting to his monthly psychotherapy appointments, once there, Mr. Williams grieved openly about his condition and tried objectively to contemplate his future. After the suicide attempt his cardiologists listened with a new seriousness to his request to have his defibrillator deactivated. They promised to explore the ethical and legal side of such acts while the psychiatrist worked with him to treat his depression. The possibility of an escape seemed to be coming within his grasp.

After several months of psychotherapy and a series of medication trials and dose adjustments, his psychiatrist agreed in writing that Mr. Williams was competent and rational. His depression had improved with treatment, and his judgment was not distorted. He understood all the relevant aspects of his medical picture, including the consequences of deactivating his defibrillator. He did not want to commit suicide; he simply wanted to be "allowed to die" naturally of his underlying disease.

His psychiatrist asked for an independent second opinion before making a final determination. After evaluating Mr. Williams, the second psychiatrist agreed that he had been given an adequate trial of medication and psychotherapy. The second psychiatrist raised the question of electroconvulsive therapy (ECT) as a treatment of last resort, but after discussing it with Mr. Williams he did not recommend it. Mr. Williams was terrified that he would be forced to endure another kind of "shock therapy," ironically so similar to the defibrillator from which he was trying to free himself. After exploring the issue directly with Mr. Williams, the psychiatrist confirmed that he was both competent and rational. In discussing whether depression was a part of the decision, he wrote, "it is a circular issue because he is depressed because of how he feels medically. While one can never know with 100 percent certainty that depression will not remit until one has exhausted trials of all medicines that are available, as well as shock treatments, we really do not have anything to indicate that this would be a remitting disorder. . . . The options for alternative antidepressant regimens including ECT have been discussed, and Mr. Williams is not interested in pursuing any further trials."

Armed with his psychiatric stamp of approval, Mr. Williams returned to his cardiologist with the request to deactivate the defibrillator so that he could die in peace. There was still one more roadblock, a formal ethics consultation to ensure that such acts were within current ethical and legal standards. Although the cardiologist might be criticized for being overly cautious, he knew that Mr. Williams would die as an indirect consequence of his actions. He wanted to be doubly sure that all bases had been covered.

I first met Mr. Williams and his wife, armed with medical records, psychiatric reports, and remarkable determination, at the end of this long road. Reading about his saga, especially what he had undergone during the last year, and seeing his diminished physical condition, my ire about a medical system out of control was clearly activated. How could he have been forced to attempt suicide before having his request taken seriously?

Yet my job was to objectively assess Mr. Williams' request from a clinical, ethical, and legal point of view and then advise both him and his cardiologist. It was a huge decision. His life and well-being literally hung in the balance. If I gave the go-ahead, his defibrillator would be deactivated and he would probably achieve his wished-for death. If I said no, he would likely live longer, but under circumstances he found untenable. How should I proceed?

First of all, the ethics and legalities of these decisions are very well established, varying little from state to state. Mentally competent patients have the right to refuse medical treatment even if it is certain that they will live with the treatment and die without it. Overriding an individual's fully informed request not to have such life-sustaining intervention, no matter what the moral justification, is not considered acceptable. The competent patient's right to refuse treatment is also extended to his right to discontinue treatment once started. This has been applied to mechanical ventilators, dialysis machines, and feeding tubes that have been started under one set of circumstances, only to be stopped when the patient's condition and wishes changed. Although there were no prior case reports of discontinuing an implantable defibrillator for a patient who wished to die, the necessary precedents were present for extending the principle.

The most challenging clinical task then became to assess Mr. Williams' mental competence to make such a decision. Was his sadness a normal response to his medical losses or had it evolved into a clinical depression that was falsely distorting his judgment? "Allowing him to die" by discontinuing a life-sustaining therapy if his request was based on an inaccurate perception of his condition would be a grave clinical error. On the other hand, forcing a suffering patient who fully understands his situation to submit to unwanted treatment adds to his agony rather than ameliorating it and borders on abuse.

After reviewing his medical records and the consultants' reports, talking with his main cardiologist, and exploring these issues with him and his wife for ninety minutes, I felt sure that that Mr. Williams was competent and rational. All reasonable standards of informed consent had been met, and he was therefore well within his rights to have his defibrillator deactivated. I reassured him and his wife that what Mr. Williams was asking for had nothing to do with suicide. In fact, we make do-not-resuscitate (DNR) decisions almost as a matter of routine for our severely ill patients. If Mr. Williams had made a DNR request, no one would have questioned his rationality, given the burden of his disease. It might even have been recommended by his physicians, given his poor prognosis and the burden of his disease. It was only because he was automatically being shocked by an advanced technological device that this question was even being asked.

Mr. Williams was both exhausted and relieved by our conversation. He hoped that he had just negotiated his final hurdle in his long struggle to have his defibrillator deactivated. I asked when he planned to have the procedure done. To my surprise, he said he was going to the cardiology office immediately after leaving our consultation. He laughed when I asked if he was sure he didn't want to think it over a while longer and reiterated that he had truly been ready a year ago.

I left the consultation room to call the cardiologist, who confirmed the plan to deactivate the device if I deemed it acceptable. On the phone, I reviewed patients' rights to discontinue life-sustaining therapy, how thoughtful Mr. Williams had appeared, and the analogy to a DNR decision. The deactivation would be a simple, noninvasive procedure. The consequences would be profound.

I went back in to see Mr. Williams and his wife and confirmed that the cardiologist was ready. We then discussed the plan for how to proceed after the deactivation. We would initiate a comfort-oriented approach. I offered to refer him to a hospice program, but he felt very connected to his current nurses and home health aides in the traditional home care system. We completed a home DNR order so that if an ambulance was called, the emergency medical technicians would not be obligated to try cardiopulmonary resuscitation. We talked about stopping any medicine and treatment that did not directly contribute to his quality of life. He preferred to continue all his medicines but wanted no more blood tests or procedures. He knew there were no guarantees that he would die easily of a sudden arrhythmia. Instead, he might have further complications that might be debilitating but not fatal. The timing was also uncertain. He might die in minutes, or it might take weeks or months. Mr. Williams was willing to accept what came.

I finally suggested that he could change his mind and have the device reactivated in the future. He smiled ironically and confirmed that he doubted that would be the case. Ordinarily there is a waiting period between the decision and the associated discontinuance of treatment, especially when there is no clinical immediacy. But in Mr. Williams' case I agreed that he had already waited more than long enough.

"Amen!" he said.

Mr. Williams saw his cardiologist later that morning. Deactivating the device was technically simple; using a remote-control device, it took only a matter of minutes, causing no added pain and requiring no invasiveness. The travel and the interview had been physically draining, but he left feeling more peaceful than he had felt in years. Although he remained physically exhausted and in pain for his last weeks, his existential agony disappeared. He patiently waited for his death. His wife remained at his side, and the aides and nurses were as attentive as always. He talked very little about death or dying; the good-byes were all implicit. His final time appeared peaceful. He sat quietly in his chair, waiting for his escape.

Fortunately, he did not have to wait long. Three weeks after the decision he was found dead. He had finally had a fatal arrhythmia. There was no sign of struggle, and the event was not dramatic. On his death certificate his demise was codified as "sudden cardiac death."

Commentary

1. *Medical technology has the potential to achieve extraordinary good as well as extraordinary harm.* Mr. Williams' life was prolonged for several years, and he was thereby able to have added time to enjoy his family and friends. What higher good can there be? Yet that same technology subsequently prolonged his dying, including a year filled mainly with agony and degradation. The possibility of such harm clearly warrants that life-sustaining technology be used with discretion. If Mr. Williams' doctors had known that it was their responsibility to discontinue his life-prolonging medical technology when it had outlived its usefulness, the damage could have been considerably lessened, if not eliminated. Physicians who help patients by using these interventions must become well versed in their responsibility to discontinue them when patients request them to because their condition or goals have changed.

Ethicists and lawyers claim that there are no significant distinctions between stopping and not starting a life-sustaining therapy, but clinicians repeatedly report that there are substantial emotional and experiential differences. This is particularly true when the act of stopping the treatment is closely followed by the patient's death. The clearest example might be taking a patient off a mechanical ventilator (breathing machine) when the patient cannot sustain breathing on his or her own. Sometimes we even have to give sedation to such patients when they begin to struggle at the very end to prevent the devastating experience of suffocation. Although we are told that such actions are ethically passive, they seem very active.

Perhaps in no other area is the technological fight for life so dramatic and successful as in cardiology, where broken hearts are restarted and nurtured every day. Deactivating Mr. Williams' defibrillator was technically simple for his cardiologist, yet it went against fundamental notions about his responsibilities. It may have been the ethically correct action, but it certainly did not feel right. Discontinuing life-sustaining treatment for patients like Mr. Williams should be difficult; after all, his death was a foreseeable consequence. However, it must not be so hard that patients have to beg for assistance or act on their own in desperation. It should be the subject of carefully constructed policies and guidelines.

2. *We must listen to and learn from those who begin to talk about the wish for death even if we feel that we cannot directly help them.* The isolation and despair that result from wishing for death but finding no one willing to take one seriously make an already untenable situation worse. By listening to such stories and trying to understand why they emerge at a particular point in time, we often can learn about avenues of helping that have nothing to do with assisting death. Sometimes the wish to die can be a signal of an emerging treatable depression or perhaps a new physical symptom that might be relieved if it is fully appreciated. It may also signal a problem in the family, such as a caregiver's fatigue or a crisis being experienced by a close relative, that might improve with a social intervention. Perhaps the patient has had a spiritual crisis while trying to understand why God has given him or her this particular burden. Exploring these crises may lead to interventions that enhance the quality of the dying process for both patient and family and are a far cry from assisting death. In the absence of open exploration the opportunity to be helpful might be lost.

Acquiescing too readily to requests for assisting death (whether by stopping a life-sustaining therapy or by more direct methods) is just as pernicious as avoiding the question. One could conceivably circumvent the entire caring process by prematurely "allowing someone to die." The opportunity to be heard, to be taken seriously as a person, and to be responded to are at the core of humane care. One must not only search for underlying causes and alternative ways to be helpful but also have an open mind to the possibility that the patient has reached the end of his or her ability and willingness to cope. One's response then may depend in part on the patient's circumstances (i.e., whether the patient is dependent on life-sustaining therapy) and in part on one's own willingness to respond to such requests (i.e., whether assisting such a patient to die lies within one's own value structure). In Mr. Williams' situation, a serious dialogue should have been started a year before his death. Much of his added desperation and despair, as well as his abortive suicide attempt, would likely have been prevented by such discussion.

3. *Suicide is defined as "the intentional taking of one's own life," but a second definition emphasizes the "destruction of the self," which makes the act generally so abhorrent.* Mr. Williams felt that his life was being destroyed by the relentless progression of his disease, and he felt that the life-sustaining technology was only prolonging his agony. Death for him became a form of self-preservation rather than self-destruction. He didn't want to die, but he preferred death to continued living under the conditions he was forced to endure. Unfortunately, because his defibrillator continued to "save" him from a sudden cardiac death, he had no escape from the nightmare that his life had become. He saw this clearly and rationally. Death was not his enemy. Continued imposed living under circumstances devoid of quality was far more pernicious and frightening.

Yet if he had not had a treatment to stop, his wish for death under otherwise identical clinical conditions would probably have been considered suicidal and, by implication, a sign of psychopathology. Any physician who took his request seriously and responded to it by helping him to die would have to act in secret, in an ethical gray zone, and in violation of laws that passively prohibit such acts. Is it any wonder that physicians tend to avoid these questions? Listening and responding to such severe suffering and exploring the wish to die are challenging enough in themselves without confounding the discussion with significant legal and ethical uncertainty.

Our language does not have a term to adequately describe the wish for death when one's personhood is being destroyed by the relentless progression of disease. People's views about when this point is reached vary widely. But the consequences of misperceiving the significance of requests for aid-in-dying under such circumstances can be devastating.

Although *suicide* is technically the correct term, its meaning confounds rather than contributes to the kind of understanding these patients deserve.

4. *Unraveling the potential contribution of depression can be challenging but usually achievable.* Mr. Williams' initial wish to die was minimized and ignored. As a result, the opportunity to find a potentially treatable depression was lost, as was the possibility of letting him stop his life-sustaining treatment when it had outlived its usefulness. When he took an overdose six months later, he was clinically depressed. It was then impossible to assess the rationality of his wish to die because depression was distorting his reasoning. Several months later, with the aid of psychotherapy and antidepressant medication, his thinking had again cleared. His mood, though far from happy, was not overwhelming his other perceptions. Unfortunately, he still wanted to die, in large measure because he understood his condition, prognosis, and treatment options so clearly.

There are no fully agreed-upon standards of rationality and competence for making these types of medical decisions. If in order to be considered rational a decision must be made without emotion or uninfluenced by factors that are out of our conscious awareness, then no decisions of consequence could meet this standard. All decisions are influenced to some degree by our feelings, our personal experience, our social context, and other factors out of our conscious awareness. Patients' decisions that go against prevailing norms are thus often disallowed. Dying patients are allowed to consent to experimental therapy in spite of its profound consequences and poor odds because these decisions reaffirm our cultural belief in the centrality of the fight for life. However, when such patients discuss the possibility of wanting to die, their rationality is questioned at every turn and unreachable standards of mental competence are proposed.

Standards of informed consent must sometimes be applied in the presence of depression, which often accompanies serious illness. Otherwise, we will further disempower those whose life and choices are already severely diminished by the consequences of their disease. The following questions were addressed in my effort to assess the rationality of Mr. Williams' request to have his life-sustaining defibrillator discontinued: (1) Did he have an accurate grasp of his condition, prognosis, and treatment options? (2) Was his request distorted by a potentially reversible mental disorder? (3) Had his request been sustained over time? (4) Did he understand the alternatives to discontinuing the defibrillator? (5) Had independent consultants assessed his competence? Once it was carefully determined that Mr. Williams' request was both rational and fully informed, our professional obligation was to respond by deactivating his defibrillator and "allowing him to die."

5. *What if Mr. Williams had wanted to die but had not had his life-sustaining therapy to discontinue?* Unfortunately, in medical ethics and law there has been excessive emphasis on methods of death and not enough on the kind of joint communication and caring that should characterize all end-of-life decision making. Stopping a patient's life-sustaining treatment, such as a defibrillator, is characterized as "allowing" that patient to die and is considered morally acceptable. Providing a prescription of barbiturates that a patient can then take on his or her own is called "assisted suicide" and is defined as a form of active "killing." Yet, clearly one could "kill" a patient by stopping his life-sustaining therapy if it was done against her or his will, under coercion, or for nefarious motives. Just as clearly, a suffering patient who had no other alternatives such as a life-sustaining treatment to stop could be "allowed to die" by means of self-administered barbiturates. The method per se does not define the morality of the act. It is defined instead by the intentions, the quality of the relationship, and the decision making of the primary actors, usually the patient, the patient's family, and the physician. Mr. Williams was "allowed to die" because he had a life-sustaining treatment to stop. Without such a possibility, his personhood might have been even more devastated in dying than it was in this sad story. We must learn to give better choices to all dying patients, no matter what their clinical circumstances, and not hide behind false distinctions and hazy lines.

References

Limits and Potential of Medical Technology

Barsky, A. J. *Worried Sick: Our Troubled Quest for Wellness.* Boston: Little, Brown, 1988.

Callahan, D. Pursuing a peaceful death. *Hastings Center Report,* July–August 1993, 33–38.

Illich, I. *Medical Nemesis,* New York: Bantam, 1976.

Mold, J. W., and H. F. Stein. The cascade effect in the clinical care of patients. *New England Journal of Medicine* 314 (1986): 512–14.

Solomon, M. Z., L. O'Donnell, B. Jennings, V. Guilfoy, S. M. Wolf, K. Nolan, R. Jackson, D. Koch-Weser, and S. Donnelley. Decisions near the end of life: Professional views on life-sustaining treatments. *American Journal of Public Health* 83 (1993): 14–23.

The SUPPORT Principal Investigators. A controlled trial to improve care for seriously ill hospitalized patients: The study to understand prognoses and preferences for outcomes and risks of treatment (SUPPORT). *Journal of the American Medical Association* 274 (1995): 1591–98.

Exploring the Wish for Death

Ackerman, F. The significance of a wish. *Hastings Center Report,* July–August 1991, 27–29.

Block, S. D., and A. Billings. Patient requests to hasten death: Evaluation and management in terminal care. *Archives of Internal Medicine* 154 (1994): 2039–47.

Gert, B., J. L. Bernat, and R. P. Mogielnicki. Distinguishing between patients' refusals and requests. *Hastings Center Report,* July–August 1994, 13–15.

Quill, T. E. Doctor, I want to die. Will you help me? *Journal of the American Medical Association* 270 (1993): 870–73.

Rie, M. A. The limits of a wish. *Hastings Center Report,* July–August 1991, 24–27.

The Language of Suicide

Brody, H. Causing, intending, and assisting death. *Journal of Clinical Ethics* 4 (1993): 112–17.

Conwell, Y., and E. D. Caine. Rational suicide and the right to die: Reality and myth. *New England Journal of Medicine* 325 (1991): 1100–1103.

Daube, D. The linguistics of suicide. *Suicide and Life-Threatening Behavior* 7 (1977): 132–82.

Quill, T. E. The ambiguity of clinical intentions. *New England Journal of Medicine* 329 (1993): 1039–40.

Quill, T. E., and R. V. Brody. "You promised me I wouldn't die like this": A bad death as a medical emergency. *Archives of Internal Medicine* 155 (1995): 1250–54.

Suicide, Depression, and Terminal Illness

Baile, W. F., J. R. DiMaggio, D. V. Schapira, and J. S. Janofsky. The request for assistance in dying: The need for psychiatric consultation. *Cancer* 72 (1993): 2786–91.

Breitbart, W. Cancer pain and suicide. In *Pain Research and Therapy*, ed. K. M. Foley et al., 399–412. New York: Raven, 1990.

Copeland, A. R. Suicide among AIDS patients. *Medicine, Science and the Law* 33 (1993): 21–28.

Harris, E. C., and B. M. Barraclough. Suicide as an outcome for medical disorders. *Medicine* 73 (1994): 281–96.

Kliban, M. G. Suicide and the hospice patient. *American Journal of Hospice Care*, March–April 1987, 15–21.

MacKenzie, T. B., and M. K. Popkin. Suicide in the medical patient. *International Journal of Psychiatry in Medicine* 17 (1987): 3–22.

Massie, M. J., P. Gagnon, and J. C. Holland. Depression and suicide in patients with cancer. *Journal of Pain and Symptom Management* 9 (1994): 325–40.

Schneiderman, E. S. Some essentials of suicide and some implications for response. In *Suicide*, ed. A. Roy, 1–16. Baltimore: Williams & Wilkins, 1986.

The Wish to Die When There Is No Life-sustaining Treatment to Discontinue

Eddy, D. M. A conversation with my mother. *Journal of the American Medical Association* 272 (1994): 179–81.

Quill, T. E. When all else fails. *Pain Forum* 4 (1995): 189–91.

Quill, T. E., S. S. Barold, and B. Sussman. Discontinuing an implantable cardioverter-defibrillator as a life-sustaining treatment. *American Journal of Cardiology* 74 (1994): 205–7.

Quill, T. E., and R. V. Brody. "You promised me I wouldn't die like this": A bad death as a medical emergency. *Archives of Internal Medicine* 155 (1995): 1250–54.

Sullivan, M. D., and S. J. Youngner. Depression, competence, and the right to refuse life saving medical treatment. *American Journal of Psychiatry* 151 (1994): 971–78.

Chapter 5

"Another Cross to Bear"

Our relationship began very slowly. Her first appointment was for a urinary-tract infection. I noticed a large scar on her arm. It was from a childhood burn; she did not want to elaborate. After several broken appointments she came in with a vaginal infection. I questioned her about sexual contacts. She allowed that her husband sometimes "messed around." She could only have contracted it from their infrequent sexual encounters. Her answers were always short and guarded, in response to the specific question, without elaboration.

Although we were close in age, we were worlds apart in terms of culture and experience. She was black and I was white. She was a nurse's aide and I was a beginning physician. She bore the scars of unstated childhood trauma, while I came from a relatively privileged background. Mrs. Johnson and Dr. Quill. Trust would be hard to develop. Perhaps we would never know each other as persons.

After several more missed appointments and another urinary-tract infection, Mrs. Johnson required hospitalization for a severe kidney infection (pyelonephritis). Since she never wanted to come into the office for a complete evaluation, this hospitalization provided my first opportunity to fully explore her medical history. She still was not eager to elaborate on the details, but the outline of her story began to be established. She was one of seven children. A sister had died from complications of diabetes, and a brother from a gunshot wound to the head. A third sibling was institutionalized, having been born with congenital syphilis. Her father, an alcoholic, had died of cirrhosis of the liver. Her mother had lived in a halfway house, suffering from unspecified mental problems for as long as she could remember. The oldest daughter, Mrs. Johnson had helped raise her younger sisters and brothers. She had held the family together since early childhood, finding the support that she lacked from her parents in the church.

Mrs. Johnson had a deep faith that God would carry her through the roughest of times. Her first profound spiritual experience had occurred when she was burned as a child. She had been hospitalized for a long time. She remembered her contacts with doctors and nurses as physically painful and psychologically distant. God had been her main companion and support, and thereafter she would always feel comforted by his presence.

Mrs. Johnson had her first child at age fifteen and was married by the time she was seventeen. She and her husband had two more children before she was twenty. She devoted herself to her children, working hard to give them a better life. As a nurse's aide she provided a warm, human touch to those in need. Her children were well behaved, and they did well in school in spite of the drugs and social chaos all around them. Her husband was another story. Although he cared about Mrs. Johnson and his family when he was sober, he had a severe drinking problem and periodically drifted into intravenous drug use. He would be gone for weeks at a time and then would return to "normal family life" as if nothing had happened. He could be quite caring during these periods and was never verbally or physically abusive, but he frequently brought back sexually transmitted diseases. Because of several associated severe pelvic infections, Mrs. Johnson had scarring around her fallopian tubes and was unable to have more children. This eventually led to a hysterectomy. When I hospitalized her for pyelonephritis, she and her husband had been separated for six months. She missed his companionship when he was not drinking or using drugs, but the price of allowing him back in her life was too high. She would now look for the support she needed in her church.

After hearing Mrs. Johnson's story, it was easier for me to tolerate her broken appointments and the distance she needed to maintain in our relationship. She had been hurt and disappointed too many times in the past. Through shared experience, perhaps trust could be established between us over time.

She returned for a follow-up appointment after her hospitalization. The infection had fully cleared. Once again the encounter was all business. Over the next year Mrs. Johnson scheduled and then missed two more appointments. Part in irritation and part out of concern, I tried to call her, but her phone had been disconnected. I subsequently learned that she had lost her job as a nurse's aide because of an absence when one of her children was sick. She had no reliable family support for emergencies, and the cost of professional childcare was prohibitive. She applied for temporary welfare to support her family but was actively looking for work. She hated being on public assistance. There would be plenty to do at home raising three children as a single parent, but she needed to work both for her self-esteem and for the added income.

I next saw Mrs. Johnson about one year later, in 1984. She was back at work as a nurse's aide. Her life had been relatively uneventful. Her children were doing well in school, remaining healthy and out of trouble. She, however, had gained thirty pounds and felt a fullness in her pelvic area. Although she had had a hysterectomy and had had no recent sexual contact with her husband or anyone else, she wondered if she might be pregnant. Since being a mother was her most meaningful activity, she thought this might be her "miracle baby"—an act of God. Perhaps they had not removed her entire uterus during her hysterectomy. As I tried to explore and gently confront her fantasy, she reported that her breasts were expelling large amounts of milk. She had to wear absorbent pads in her bra and change them frequently. I was initially skeptical, but when I examined her breasts, the milk was indeed flowing. She looked at me, expectant and proud. When I examined her internally, I felt a fullness but no enlarged uterus.

"What do you think?" she asked.

"I am not sure what to think. I doubt that you are pregnant, given your hysterectomy, but we will have to pursue all possibilities, from pregnancy to a hormonal imbalance to some kind of tumor. I would like to schedule some blood tests and an ultrasound of your pelvic area."

"I feel exactly the way I did when I was pregnant," she said with a smile. "I think you are wrong."

We made an appointment to meet as soon as the results were in. The ultrasound was normal. The fullness I had identified had been from postsurgical scarring and from weight gain. Her blood tests showed an elevated level of prolactin, a hormone made by the pituitary gland that stimulates the breasts to make milk. Her pregnancy test was negative, as were the other tests of hormonal function. Mrs. Johnson was very disappointed as well as skeptical about the results. Even though her life as a single parent of three young children was at times exhausting and overwhelming, she would have loved another baby. Newborns were so wonderfully giving and accepting.

"How sure are you that I am not pregnant?"

"Unfortunately, I am very sure."

"I'm not sure that I believe you."

"I know you are very disappointed."

Excessive prolactin often comes from a growth in the pituitary gland known as an adenoma. It is not a cancer, but because it lies in a very small, enclosed space, it can cause problems if it grows beyond a tiny size. Untreated, such adenomas can impair vision and put pressure on other structures at the base of the brain. A new, relatively noninvasive surgery is available to shrink the tumor if it gets large enough to create trouble. If it is small, it can be followed clinically, and the galactorrhea (milk secretion by the breasts) can be suppressed by medicine that impedes prolactin production and release. I recommended a CT scan of the brain to determine the tumor's size, along with medication to decrease the galactorrhea. Mrs. Johnson listened carefully, but she was not ready to undertake treatment or further tests. Since the situation was not overly urgent or dangerous, I did not push her for an immediate decision. Mrs. Johnson needed to be in charge of what happened to her body, and efforts to control or coerce her were met with outright resistance. She would make decisions independently, on her own terms, when she was ready.

She came to her next two appointments with questions arising from reading she had done about pituitary adenomas. She had verified what I had told her in several independent sources. She then agreed to a CT scan, which showed a tiny microadenoma in her pituitary gland. Its small size was reassuring. Surgery would not be needed, and we could take our time in the decision making without putting her at risk. Medicine was available to suppress the galactorrhea, but not taking it was also a viable option, providing she could tolerate the milk secretion. She did not want any treatment that was not absolutely necessary. We would meet every three months to check her exam and the hormone levels and every six months to do visual field testing. It was a plan we both were comfortable with.

During the next two years Mrs. Johnson came to most of her regularly scheduled appointments. We would always begin by checking the status of her hormone levels, the amount of galactorrhea, and any visual changes she was experiencing. Once she developed headaches that necessitated repeatedly checking the size of her adenoma. She also tried several short courses of bromocryptine, the drug used to suppress prolactin production. Our conversation gradually broadened to include her life at home with her family and at work. She and her husband had separated and then gotten back together several more times. It was helpful to have him around the house when he wasn't drinking but very painful when he would disappear again. She eventually stopped allowing him to return even when he was sober. Her church believed that drugs and alcohol were evil, incompatible with a Christian life. Their advice was to give him up unless he could commit to living a life without this kind of sin.

Early in 1987 she came in for a visit visibly upset. We skipped the traditional medical exchange and went directly to what was bothering her. Her youngest daughter, the "baby" for whom she had had aspirations of college and a different kind of life, had become pregnant at age fifteen. Having been through teenage pregnancy herself, she knew that it made finding a way out of poverty much more difficult. Her oldest daughter, then nineteen, already had two children and had not finished high school. She saw the cycle continuing with no escape. She felt like a failure as a mother. She had given her daughters clear information about how to avoid getting pregnant: "If not abstinence, then at least use protection!" Somehow the message had not gotten through. She loved the grandchildren and spent considerable time helping her children to raise them. But she also knew that her own children's potential would now be much more limited than if they had waited to complete their own schooling before having children. Once she worked through her grief and disappointment, she acknowledged that having all the generations under one roof gave life a richness and excitement.

I met Mr. Johnson several times in the early 1980s. Usually these brief encounters occurred when he and his wife needed simultaneous treatment for a sexually transmitted infection so that they wouldn't pass it back and forth. He felt guilty about his drinking, his drug use, and the associated promiscuity, but somehow he couldn't stop. He usually became infected while on a binge, and then he couldn't remember when or from whom he had contracted the disease. Although Mr. Johnson was very engaging and personable, I found his lack of personal responsibility toward his wife frustrating.

I had not seen him in over four years when he surfaced in 1988 with an infection in his knee caused by an unusual fungus. He also had yeast growing in his throat, raising the specter of an underlying infection with human immunodeficiency virus (HIV). He was at high risk because of his intravenous drug use, to say nothing of his anonymous sexual contacts. He consented to HIV testing, which confirmed that he was infected. Since so many of his drug-using friends already had been diagnosed with HIV, the news was not unexpected. He gave his permission to share the information with his wife. Since their sexual contact had been very infrequent in the past five years, we were both hopeful that she had not been infected.

Mrs. Johnson made an appointment for "pretest counseling," during which the implications of the test could be explored before it was actually performed. This provided an opportunity to discuss the meaning of the disease, explore potential treatment options, clarify misconceptions, and answer questions. She confirmed that she and her husband had had sexual intercourse only rarely but that they had not used condoms. She had had no other sexual partners since adolescence. She had never used intravenous drugs or had any blood transfusions. I explained the distinction between HIV (the early infection with the virus, which lasts for many years, during which the patient is relatively free from medical problems) and AIDS (the later stage, during which the patient is much more subject to opportunistic infections and complications). She understood the difference but called both phases AIDS, which is common. When I asked her what it would mean if she were infected, she responded, "I don't know, but I don't think God would do this to me." Given the central role that faith played in her life, this response left me unsettled, but we agreed to proceed with testing anyway. An appointment was scheduled to discuss the results, positive or negative. I suggested that she might want to have a family member with her, but she preferred to hear the results alone.

The test showed that she was infected with HIV. I found the report in the middle of a mountain of papers. I felt numb, and I couldn't concentrate, saddened for her as a person. It also brought home to me the realization that this epidemic was reaching people in all walks of life. I began to dread our upcoming visit, uncertain about how she would respond. I feared that this could shake the foundations of her faith and her sense of who she was. I shared my concerns with one of my physician partners so that I would be better prepared to respond to Mrs. Johnson without simultaneously working through my own grief. How could this happen to Mrs. Johnson, who had overcome so much and worked so hard? How many other of our patients and friends must be latently infected with HIV? There is nothing fair about this disease.

What follows is an unedited transcript of the first minutes of our meeting:

Mrs. Johnson: Is it bad?

Dr. Quill: I'm afraid it is.

Mrs. Johnson: Oh no, Dr. Quill, oh my God!

Dr. Quill: I was shocked too.

Mrs. Johnson: Oh God! Oh Lord have mercy! Oh God, don't tell me that! Oh Lord have mercy! Oh my God! Oh my God, no, Dr. Quill! Oh God! Oh no! Please don't do it again! Please don't tell me that! Oh my God! Oh my children! Oh Lord have mercy! Oh God, why did He do this to me? Why did He do this to me? Why did He do this to me, Dr. Quill? Oh Lord have mercy! Oh my God, Jesus!

Dr. Quill: You're still alright at this point, okay?

Mrs. Johnson: You don't know how long I've had it, Dr. Quill?

Dr. Quill: I don't know.

Mrs. Johnson: I can't sit. [*She paces around room.*]

Dr. Quill: It's okay. [*I stand up.*]

Mrs. Johnson: Why did He do this to me? Why? What have I done to him? Why does He do this to me? Why? Why? Oh Lord! What am I going to do with all of my children? I won't be able to see my grandchildren. I just had another grandbaby. I won't ever be able to see . . . I won't live to see the baby. I won't be able to get up off my chair. Oh, Dr. Quill, I don't know what to do. Oh God, I don't know what to do! My son-in-law is not going to let the kids come over.

Dr. Quill: First thing we have to do is learn as much as we can about it, because right now you are okay.

Mrs. Johnson: I don't even have a future. Everything I know is that you gonna die anytime. What is there to do? What if I'm a walking time bomb? People will be scared to even touch me or say anything to me.

Dr. Quill: No, that's not so.

Mrs. Johnson: Yes they will, 'cause I feel that way about people. You don't know what to say to them and what to do. Oh God!

Dr. Quill: What we have to do is learn some things about it . . . even though it's scary it may not be as scary as you think. Okay?

Mrs. Johnson: Oh my God! Oh my God! I hate him! I hate him! I hate the ground he walks on! I hate him, Dr. Quill! I hate him! He gave this to me. I hate him! He took my life away from me! I have been robbed. I feel as if I have been robbed of a future. I don't have nothing.

Dr. Quill: There is a future for you.

Mrs. Johnson: They don't even have a cure for me.

Dr. Quill: There's a lot of work going on right now, and you can have the infection for a long time before you get sick. There is a lot of research going on.

Mrs. Johnson: I read about it. I have a friend with it. I went over to the university. . . . Since you told him he had AIDS, he has been at my house and I feel so sorry for him. I was being nice to him. Oh my God, my God! It just doesn't pay to be nice! It doesn't! What do you get out of it?

Dr. Quill: Neither you nor he knew that there was a risk back then.

Mrs. Johnson: Another cross to bear.

Dr. Quill: You never did anything wrong.

Mrs. Johnson: What am I going to tell my children when they are old enough to tell them?

Dr. Quill: Before you tell them anything, you are going to learn a lot about this.

Mrs. Johnson: I can't go home! I can't even stay here! I'm so scared! Oh my God! I knew that you were going to tell me this! I always liked you. I didn't want you to tell me this. Oh God! I don't know if I can deal with this. I don't know, Dr. Quill, if I can deal with this.

Dr. Quill: You've worked through this before. It's going to be hard, but it may not be as bad as you think. Okay? I think what you have to do . . .

Mrs. Johnson: I got my church, Dr. Quill. I can't let them see me like that. I can't do it. I would rather . . . because I can't let our church see me like this. They mean a lot to me. Oh, Dr. Quill, and my daughter. Oh, I won't see my daughter and my baby.

Dr. Quill: You're still the same person. Okay?

Mrs. Johnson: Why is He doing this to me?

Dr. Quill: I don't know. You are still the same person. What we have to do is eventually learn as much as you can about this. The odds are that you are going to stay healthy for a long time. Okay? You are still very healthy right now.

Mrs. Johnson: What you telling me? I still have a chance to beat it? Can I beat it?

Dr. Quill: I think that is possible.

Mrs. Johnson: How can you be sure when you don't even know what the cure is for it?

Dr. Quill: A couple of things, okay? We don't think you've had this very long; a couple of years at the most. Alright. A lot of people believe that the virus can stay around for many years before it produces many problems. Sometimes six or eight years. There is a lot of research going on now to try to find ways to treat it.

Mrs. Johnson: Oh God, Lord Jesus!

Dr. Quill: You may have a lot of time before we have to deal with this. I think the first thing we have to do is probably get some further blood tests. We should because it's such a surprise for you and for me that you have it, even though we think we know how you got it. We maybe should repeat it to be 100 percent, 1,000 percent sure, even though they repeat it once. I think that's wise to do because the only way that you could have gotten it is from your husband. I think we ought to repeat it even though we know that it is probably true.

Mrs. Johnson: I don't know how I can live with myself. . . . In my bed right now. I don't like him, Dr. Quill. I don't even want to stand by him. I won't even stay with him. I won't. Why must I pay for his sins? Why?

Dr. Quill: There's nothing fair about it.

Mrs. Johnson: My children.

Dr. Quill: It's very scary. Also, there are a lot of things we can do.

Mrs. Johnson: Oh Lord have mercy. Then I have the pituitary thing.

Dr. Quill: Like your pituitary tumor, it has been there for years. It doesn't . . .

Mrs. Johnson: It's not the same.

Dr. Quill: No, it's not the same thing. If the tumor gets worse, we know what the treatment is.

Mrs. Johnson: It's not the same. It can't be cured! You talking about something they never came up with, never came up with a cure for. I've got nothing. All they can do is just treat whatever comes along, like a cold, or pneumonia, stuff like that—that's all.

Dr. Quill: That's right. But right now there are millions and millions of dollars being poured into research and that's what we have to hope for.

Mrs. Johnson: It doesn't make me feel good.

Dr. Quill: I wish I had something more clear to tell you, but I think there are a lot of folks who are in the same shoes that you're in and they are all hoping. They are figuring out ways to cope. That's what we have to figure out.

Mrs. Johnson: Dr. Quill, will you still be my doctor?

Dr. Quill: Absolutely, I will.

Mrs. Johnson: You promise?

Dr. Quill: Absolutely. We'll meet very regularly so we know what's going on.

Mrs. Johnson: Okay, alright. I'm so scared. I don't want to die. I don't want to die, Dr. Quill, not yet. I know I got to die, but I don't want to die.[1]

I fought back my own tears until she asked if I was going to abandon her because she was infected. I reassured her that we were in this together. Luckily, we had a shared history, so she trusted my responses and did not feel completely alone as she tried to grasp the meaning of this devastating news.

During the encounter, Mrs. Johnson seemed to fall into a black hole. "I don't even have a future. Everything I know is that you gonna die anytime. What is there to do? What if I'm a walking time bomb? People will be scared to even touch me or say anything to me." I clumsily tried to help her find boundaries to her hopelessness and despair when none were apparent. This search for edges was as much for me as it was for her, for it is very hard to "be with" such free-floating terror without trying to limit it. The transcript does not do justice to the emotional and physical intensity of the encounter—the crying, yelling, pacing, and hugging. It was well outside of my usual experience. I believe, however, that Mrs. Johnson was outwardly demonstrating what most persons experience on the inside when they are faced with devastating news.

In the midst of her intense emotional outpouring Mrs. Johnson raised several fundamental questions: (1) Would I still be her doctor (would she be alone, or abandoned)? (2) How contagious (repulsive) was she? (3) Was she still the same person? (4) When and how was she going to die? (5) How could she tell her family, friends, and church? Although there were no simple answers, together we struggled to find some shape and definition to the problem. We spent the final ten min-

---

1. Mrs. Johnson gave me permission to tape our visit. She subsequently said that I could use the transcript and tape to teach how to deliver bad news as humanely as possible. My wife and I wrote a paper on this topic that included this narrative: T. E. Quill and P. Townsend, Delivering bad news: Delivery, dialogue, and dilemmas, *Archives of Internal Medicine* 151 (1991): 463–68.

utes of the encounter making a concrete plan for her immediate future. Where was she going from the office? Who would she go to for support? How would she tell her oldest child, who already knew that her father was infected and also knew about the purpose of our visit that day? I was somewhat afraid that she might take her life rather than face her radically altered future, especially if her children or her church were unsupportive. She reassured me that she was not going to kill herself and that her oldest daughter would understand and be supportive. I planned to talk with her by phone the next day; we would meet face to face several days later.

I was emotionally exhausted after Mrs. Johnson left. The devastating power of bad news had penetrated my defenses as well as hers. I again sat down with one of my partners to get some support and perspective and then went through the motions of doing my work for the remainder of the day. I went home knowing that I too had been permanently altered by the encounter; and I understood better than ever before the power of a diagnosis to transform the life of the person who receives it.

Mrs. Johnson sounded more integrated on the phone the next day. Her daughter had been supportive, and she was reading several lay brochures about HIV. I invited her to bring questions, as well as any family members she wished, to our next scheduled visit. I felt reassured and somewhat surprised by how optimistic she sounded. Perhaps the intense outward display of emotion was cultural—a natural beginning to her grieving process. When, however, she canceled her appointment later in the week, I again became worried. I called her at home. She explained that she was still learning about the disease and would be ready to see me in a few weeks, when she had had a chance to better formulate her questions. She sounded activated and engaged; she was finding her own path through this illness as she had found her way through so many challenges in the past.

When I saw her two weeks later, she had made considerable progress toward coming to grips with her disease. She had told all three of her children, along with several other relatives. They were all accepting and more knowledgeable than she had expected. A more detailed physical examination showed her condition to be normal except for a small amount of oral thrush. She agreed to testing to discover the level of her helper lymphocytes (the CD4 count), which is the best laboratory marker of vulnerability and prognosis.

Her CD4 count was lower than normal (400) but not in the range where more dangerous infections begin to occur (below 200). I recommended that she start zivirodine (AZT), a drug believed to delay the progression from latent HIV infection to AIDS if it is started when the CD4 count falls below 500. Mrs. Johnson was reluctant. She had seen persons dying with AIDS who had taken AZT in the past and wondered if the drug might have precipitated their downhill course. But more important, she wanted to live her life normally, as if she were uninfected. She knew that she should avoid all sexual contact and that her blood was contagious, but otherwise she didn't want to think about the infection unless it was absolutely necessary. Taking preventive medicine three times every day would be a constant reminder that she was ill and, in her eyes, more detrimental than helpful. She preferred to put her fate in the hands of the Lord. I hoped that eventually she would use medicine to supplement the healing power of her faith, but she remained steadfast in her desire to avoid AZT or any treatment directed against the HIV.

Mrs. Johnson's faith in God remained a central sustaining factor, but she never informed her minister or any members of her church about her infection. She had seen others with HIV be shunned by the church and had listened to sermons villifying the infection as part of God's punishment for an immoral lifestyle. According to her minister, there were no innocent victims. She refused to risk losing the support and sustenance of her church by sharing her secret. She never fully understood why God had given her this "cross to bear," but she appeared to accept it with grace and humility. The outward rage she had felt upon first hearing the news dissipated, and she found solace in the mystery of God's master plan. I offered to meet with her minister or to help her find another pastor who was more knowledgeable about HIV, but she declined. She was much more forgiving and accepting of her church's shortcomings than I could be.

Except for a few relatively routine respiratory infections, Mrs. Johnson's health remained stable over the next two years. In 1990, however, her CD4 count fell below 200, marking the transition from HIV to AIDS and heralding a more ominous phase of her illness. AZT and other drugs that reduce the viral burden are even more effective in preventing complications during this phase, but she remained adamant in her refusal to take them. She was still leading a normal life and wanted to ignore her illness for as long as possible. She didn't deny that she had the infection; she simply didn't want to think about it. If her time was limited, she wanted to focus her energy on her children, her grandchildren, and her church.

Mrs. Johnson was now at risk for other potentially preventable infections. Perhaps she could take advantage of these treatments even if she did not want to take AZT. She did agree to a monthly inhalation of pentamidine to prevent pneumocystis pneumonia, one of the more dangerous opportunistic infections associated with AIDS. She agreed to do this in part because the treatment was not daily but also because it was not aimed explicitly at the HIV itself. We kept searching for ways that she could benefit from proven treatments without violating what she needed to do to maintain her personal integrity.

Over the next two years Mrs. Johnson was hospitalized five times with opportunistic infections, and she was treated on an outpatient basis for several additional complications. She would usually wait until the last minute to come in; several times she almost died from infections that might have been more easily treated if we had an earlier start. She knew these delays were dangerous. I repeatedly reminded her, without browbeating, that she was playing with fire. She did not have a death wish, but she hated the prospect of being sick and dependent and hoped to postpone it for as long as possible.

During one of these hospitalizations Mrs. Johnson developed very low blood pressure from an infection with a pneumococcal bacteria in her blood stream and had to be admitted to the intensive care unit. She rapidly recovered, but with each infection she was becoming more dangerously ill. The length of time between problems was also diminishing. She was losing weight and had recurrent episodes of shingles (a painful infection of the skin caused by the chickenpox virus).

Since Mrs. Johnson's quality of life was declining, we needed to address a different set of questions about her future care in order to make it as humane as possible. The first question was about cardiopulmonary resuscitation. If she deteriorated to the point that she could no longer breathe on her own, or her heart stopped beating effectively, would she want us to use cardiopulmonary resuscitation to try to revive her? Given her deteriorating medical condition and her desire to be as unencumbered as possible by medical intervention, she clearly didn't want this treatment. Antibiotics, fluids, and other noninvasive treatments would be used as indicated, but no extraordinary or invasive measures would be employed.

We also discussed what treatment she would want if she lost the ability to speak for herself. Although everyone should complete such advance directives, persons with AIDS have a particularly grim prospect of potentially developing AIDS dementia. From the outset, Mrs. Johnson had expressed a fear about such an end ("I can't let them see me like that!"), and she wished to minimize the possibility. We talked about stopping all treatments, including antibiotics for infection and fluids for dehydration, if she became permanently demented or otherwise mentally impaired. She wanted me to make decisions based on her directive; she did not want to place that burden on her children. I agreed, but asked that she complete a living will so that her wishes were clearly expressed. This would protect her as well as me. We hoped we would never need it.

Mrs. Johnson and I had grown much closer over the past several years. I looked forward to her visits, although they were usually both medically and personally challenging. We now knew each other as persons, and our conversations were wide ranging, with few inhibitions. I worried about how the next phase of her illness might unfold. Perhaps her strategy of partial denial of the illness and its prognosis was prudent.

Six months later Mrs. Johnson began to have some trouble with her equilibrium and her memory. It was very subtle at first but then became undeniable. She initially refused a formal neurological evaluation. With the help of her children, I eventually convinced her to look for a potentially treatable cause. A CT scan of Mrs. Johnson's head showed brain atrophy out of proportion to her age, and a subsequent spinal tap revealed excess protein in the fluid surrounding her brain. Cultures, stains, and immunological studies of her spinal fluid did not yield a clear diagnosis. We feared that she was in the first stages of irreversible brain degeneration, which can accompany AIDS. With the help of nurses and home health aides from the visiting nurse service, she was initially able to stay home with her family. Mrs. Johnson's confusion increased rapidly, such that she required supervision around the clock. Her family supports began to fall apart under the burden of her constant care, so arrangements were made to admit her to the hospital, where we would try to improve the quality of her life, if not lengthen it.

In the hospital Mrs. Johnson's level of conscious awareness waxed and waned. Sometimes she was lethargic and appeared to be hallucinating. At other times she was quite lucid, somewhat able to comprehend her situation. Her coordination was abnormal, and she couldn't walk without the constant assistance of two people. Her ability to recall recent events or to retain numbers was almost completely absent. In a clear moment she consented to a magnetic resonance scan (MRI) of her brain and to a spinal tap. Since I was unsure about her capacity to give consent, I also discussed the plan with her daughter, who agreed on her mother's behalf. We would look for anything that might improve her mother's condition without adding unnecessarily to her suffering. Unfortunately, the MRI scan showed further atrophy of her brain, with degeneration in the deeper structures. Her spinal tap showed a higher level of abnormal protein but no reversible infection. Her deterioration was due to an AIDS-related dementia. Mrs. Johnson's future looked grim; she had developed the type of deterioration she feared most. The only bright spot was that she was probably so confused that she would not be aware of her worsening condition.

I discussed Mrs. Johnson's condition with her oldest daughter, who, in turn, communicated with the rest of the family. The only intervention that might possibly slow the progression of her mental deterioration was the drug AZT, and Mrs. Johnson had been adamant about avoiding it while she was mentally competent. I didn't think that we should override her wishes now that she had lost the ability to say no, but I was uncomfortable about making the decision without the family's input. Her daughter agreed with me. I recommended to the family that we pursue a comfort-oriented approach, using only interventions that would directly contribute to her quality of life. By this time they trusted me and had seen enough of their mother's anguish when she was at home to agree with this recommendation. I also suggested that we refrain from using further diagnostic procedures or antibiotics for future infections, instead suppressing her fever with acetaminophen or aspirin and sedating her when she was agitated. Pain would be treated with morphine. Here again, they found it reassuring that all medical interventions would be geared to improving Mrs. Johnson's quality of life. We explored whether the family could manage Mrs. Johnson's care at home with the assistance of a hospice program. Having already spent several months at home unsuccessfully trying to manage a deteriorating situation, they declined.

Mrs. Johnson was transferred to a long-term-care floor in our hospital and was treated according to a comfort-care philosophy. Family members visited her daily. It was painful for them to watch their mother's mental function deteriorate as she progressively lost control of her mind and her bodily functions. Although Mrs. Johnson got the best possible care under the circumstances, her mental and physical disintegration was agonizing toward the end. I hope she was unaware of her condition over the last month and that the caring presence of her family, the nursing staff, and the nurses aides somehow penetrated her confusion. She was never visited by the members of her church, who remained ignorant about her condition and her suffering. Fortunately,

Mrs. Johnson's faith was internal and unshakable. There was no doubt in her mind that she had led the best life she could given her circumstances. She would be going to a better place when she died.

Mrs. Johnson developed fever, shaking chills, and very low blood pressure about one month later. Instead of our usual diagnostic tests, cultures, antibiotics, and intravenous fluids, we suppressed her fever with acetaminophen and the shaking chills with morphine. In the absence of our medical armamentarium, her depressed immune system was no match for the infection; she died relatively peacefully within approximately twelve hours with her daughters at her side. We were all relieved that her final ordeal was over, and she was finally set free from this life, which had been so bittersweet.

Mr. Johnson survived his wife by one year. He was remorseful about causing her infection and genuinely grieved her death. He continued periodically to abuse alcohol and intravenous drugs but also took AZT and other medicines to prevent opportunistic infections. He spent most of his last year in the hospital under my care, fighting a vigorous medical battle against some of the advanced complications of AIDS, including weight loss, diarrhea, liver obstruction, fungal infections, and recurrent pneumocystis pneumonia. He too died of an overwhelming infection. His death, however, was marked by an all-out fight to prolong his life, including antibiotics, fluids, drugs to raise his blood pressure, mechanical breathing machines, and repeated electrical shocks to his heart at the very end. The contrast in the ways that Mr. and Mrs. Johnson lived and died is both striking and unsettling. Part of our privilege and our burden as physicians is to participate in and bear witness to such divergent but intersecting life stories.

Commentary

1. *Joining in partnership with patients allows medicine's power to be used in a personalized way.* Like many patients, Mrs. Johnson needed to be in charge of her own medical care and to make decisions consistent with

her beliefs and values. Patients know best about their own experience, values, and personal histories, while physicians' special knowledge is mainly about medical matters. From this perspective, medical transactions become a sharing of expertise. Personalized decisions cannot be made without knowledge about both sides of the equation. A middle ground between medical recommendations and patient preferences can almost always be found through a process of mutually informing one another, seeking common ground, and then explicitly negotiating the remaining differences. Such partnerships require mutual trust, a willingness to be flexible, and curiosity about human differences.

For Mrs. Johnson and myself, trust came slowly. In addition to the usual barriers created by differences in race, sex, and socioeconomic status, she had had very negative medical experiences when she was severely burned as a child. By facing her medical problems together, we gradually came to know each other. The flexibility I demonstrated when treating her pituitary adenoma provided a solid foundation for the time when we subsequently had to face the more challenging dilemmas posed by her HIV infection. She believed not only that I would fully inform her about the medical options and my recommendations but also that I would respect her as the ultimate decision maker. She knew that reaching conclusions that did not follow my recommendations would not compromise her subsequent care or lessen my concern about her. The more I learned about the many "crosses" she had had to bear throughout her life, the more I admired and respected her as a person. Since she would experience both the benefits and the burdens of our medical interventions, final decisions should clearly be hers to make.

2. *Denial about one's illness can be both a blessing and a curse.* If denial prohibits a person from confronting important medical and personal decisions, then it can be very harmful. However, if it allows one to keep devastating illness out of conscious awareness so that one can focus on other matters, denial can sometimes be both helpful and healthy. The psychic task of those facing severe illness is formidable. Some patients immerse themselves in their illness, becoming experts and indepen-

dently ensuring that they are getting the best of treatments. Others deny the illness in its totality, pretending to themselves and others that they are unaffected. Most, like Mrs. Johnson, choose somewhere in the middle ground, a mix of immersion and denial. Mrs. Johnson had no doubt that she was infected with HIV, but she chose not to talk about it very often. In order to avoid the potential prejudices and stereotypes of her minister and the members of her church, she refused to tell them. She devoted most of her thoughts, energies, and time to the care of her children and grandchildren. She would deal with her illness when and if she had to.

The only area of significant disagreement between us concerned the use of AZT to counteract the HIV. I thought it might delay the transition from HIV to AIDS and lessen the number and severity of complications. From her vantage point, it would be a thrice-daily reminder of her vulnerability to an incurable illness. Since AZT has subsequently proven to be less effective in the early stages than had been originally hoped, her initial decision even made some sense from a medical perspective. Her moderate level of denial allowed her to make the most of the six years from her diagnosis to her death. She faced medical problems and made decisions when it was immediately imperative. It was not always the approach I recommended, but it worked reasonably well for her.

3. *I have learned more about spirituality in caring for terminally ill patients than in any other aspect of my life.* The struggle between life and death creates an openness and immediacy to comprehending what it means to be human, what one's life has meant, and whether there is an afterlife. It is not a simple or uniform experience. A well-developed sense of spirituality and religion can often be a source of strength through one's illness and ultimate death. Yet Mrs. Johnson had an illness tainted with stigma and prejudice in her church. She therefore kept it secret from her minister and parishioners for fear of being judged and even shunned. This might have led to bitterness and even a questioning of her faith, but Mrs. Johnson's belief in a beneficent, omnipotent God did not falter. Although she never fully understood why God had

given her this particular burden, she bore it as best she could. Mrs. Johnson was afraid of dying in a way that would be humiliating for her and her family, but she was not afraid of death per se. She had a clear, sustaining vision of life after death.

Many persons with strong spiritual convictions prefer to put their faith more in God rather than in medicine when they get sick. "If it is God's will, then it is my duty to follow." When such persons have an illness for which we have effective medical treatment, we then should make every effort to combine resources. Usually common ground is found in an approach in which Western medicine and spiritualism supplement each other. Since a positive, hopeful attitude probably enhances the functioning of the immune system, there can even be "scientific" explanations for the effectiveness of combined approaches (for those who need such corroboration). Although Mrs. Johnson rejected the combined approach with regard to AZT, she did allow the use of traditional medical treatments when she developed other acute infections. In that setting, choosing medical treatment did not constitute a refusal to accept God's will but seemed to be an acceptable extension of His armamentarium. At the end, we used medical interventions to ease her physical suffering, while her family found considerable spiritual comfort in the knowledge that she believed she was leaving this life for a better place.

4. *Delivering bad news is one of our biggest challenges as physicians.* As physicians, we give patients bad news almost every day, yet we receive little training about how to do it well. When a diagnostic test, such as screening for HIV, is being contemplated, the doctor and patient can often get an idea about its potential meaning by discussing it in a hypothetical sense. In my discussion with Mrs. Johnson, she said that she "didn't think that God would do this to me." Since I knew her strong belief in God's beneficence, this was a potentially ominous reflection. This diagnosis had the potential to threaten her faith and, in doing so, to disrupt the foundation of how she made sense out of life.

Mrs. Johnson was shaken to her core during our initial conversation, reflecting the devastating potential of bad medical news. Sometimes the brain simply shuts down, leaving patients numb and overwhelmed. Others immediately ask hundreds of questions but remember few answers. When people are asked in retrospect what they would like when they receive bad news, they report wanting more information so that they can make sense out of their experience. Yet most people are initially too overwhelmed to absorb anything beyond the basic outline of the problem and the plan, so the detailed exploration of the disease and treatment options often has to wait. The clinician's challenge is to go slowly, allowing the patient to control the depth and focus of the interaction as much as possible. The primary goals of an initial encounter include achieving a common perception of the problem, addressing immediate medical risks, responding to pressing discomforts, ensuring a basic plan for follow-up, and, above all, minimizing isolation and aloneness. Usually, detailed information can be integrated over time, so the patient has some time to comprehend his or her changed circumstances before making major medical decisions with significant personal consequences.

References

Partnerships

Brody, D. S., S. M. Miller, C. E. Lerman, D. G. Smith, and G. C. Caputo. Patient perception of involvement in medical care: Relationship to illness attitudes and outcomes. *Journal of General Internal Medicine* 4 (1989): 506–11.

Emanuel, E. J., and L. L. Emanuel. Four models of the physician-patient relationship. *Journal of the American Medical Association* 267 (1992): 2221–26.

Greenfield, S., S. H. Kaplan, J. E. Ware Jr., E. M. Yano, and H. J. Frank. Patients' participation in medical care: Effects on blood sugar control and quality of life in diabetes. *Journal of General Internal Medicine* 3 (1988): 448–57.

Kaplan, S. H., S. Greenfield, and J. E. Ware Jr. Assessing the effects of physician-patient interactions on the outcomes of chronic disease. *Medical Care* 27 (1989): S110–27.

Lidz, C. W., P. S. Appelbaum, and A. Meisel. Two models of implementing informed consent. *Archives of Internal Medicine* 148 (1988): 1385–89.

May, W. F. Code, covenant, contract, or philanthropy. *Hastings Center Report,* December 1975, 29–38.

Novack, D. H. Therapeutic aspects of the clinical encounter. *Journal of General Internal Medicine* 2 (1987): 346–55.

Quill, T. E. Partnerships in patient care: A contractual approach. *Annals of Internal Medicine* 98 (1983): 228–34.

Siegler, M. The physician-patient accommodation: A central event in clinical medicine. *Archives of Internal Medicine* 142 (1982): 1899–902.

Veatch, R. M. Models for ethical medicine in a revolutionary age: What physician-patient roles foster the most ethical relationship? *Hastings Center Report,* June 1972, 5–7.

Yarmolinsky, A. Supporting the patient. *New England Journal of Medicine* 332 (1995): 602–3.

Denial

Ness, D. E., and J. Ende. Denial in the medical interview: Recognition and management. *Journal of the American Medical Association* 272 (1994): 1777–81.

Quill, T. E. Recognizing and adjusting to barriers in doctor-patient communication. *Annals of Internal Medicine* 111 (1989): 51–57.

Spirituality

Aries, P. *The Hour of Our Death.* New York: Oxford University Press, 1991.

Branch, W. T., and A. L. Suchman. Meaningful experiences in medicine. *American Journal of Medicine* 88 (1990): 56–59.

Byock, I. Growth: The essence of hospice. *American Journal of Hospice Care* 3 (1986): 16–21.

Callanan, M., and P. Kelly. *Final Gifts.* New York: Poseidon, 1992.

Frankl, V. E. *Man's Search for Meaning.* Rev ed. New York: Washington Square, 1984.

Grey, A. The spiritual component of palliative care. *Palliative Medicine* 8 (1994): 215–21.

Matthews, D. A., A. L. Suchman, and W. T. Branch. Making "connexions": Enhancing the therapeutic potential of patient-clinician relationships. *Annals of Internal Medicine* 118 (1993): 973–77.

Mermann, A. C. Spiritual aspects of death and dying. *Yale Journal of Biology and Medicine* 65 (1992): 137–42.

Bad News

Buckman, R., and Y. Kason. *How to Break Bad News: A Guide for Health Care Professionals.* Baltimore: Johns Hopkins University Press, 1992.

Derdiarian, A. K. Informational needs of recently diagnosed cancer patients. *Nursing Research* 35 (1986): 276–81.

Faulkner, A., P. Maguire, and C. Regnard. Breaking bad news—a flow diagram. *Palliative Medicine* 8 (1994): 145–51.

Girgis, A., and R. W. Sanson-Fisher. Breaking bad news: Consensus guidelines for medical practitioners. *Journal of Clinical Oncology* 13 (1995): 2449–56.

Quill, T. E., and P. Townsend. Bad news: Delivery, dialogue, and dilemmas. *Archives of Internal Medicine* 151 (1991): 463–68.

Chapter 6

Three Strikes and You're Out

I WAS BORN ON Adolph Hitler's last birthday alive: April 20, 1945. I am not sure I can exactly find the words to explain why that is significant, other than the fact that I know I am not his reincarnation. I thought this would be the first line in my book." John made this surprising revelation in an interview shortly before he died. The notion that this Jewish man born on the heels of the Holocaust would begin his life story this way might seem shocking. But John was not a simple man. His life was filled with contradiction and contrast.

When I first met him in the early 1980s, John was a broadcaster and political analyst for a local television station. He filled his life with an endless series of articles and presentations, working in frenetic bursts around deadlines alternating with long periods of procrastination and aimlessness. He was strong-willed and opinionated, a perfectionist as critical of himself as he was of everyone else. His work was highly respected, but working with him was a challenge. His temper would flare up without warning, and he would vent his considerable rage on those around him. His political interviews were entertaining; he would keep the interviewee on edge and off balance, uncertain what he might ask next.

John was extremely bright and enthusiastic. He researched his topics thoroughly, and he had a reputation for being knowledgeable and uniquely insightful about the local political scene. A World War II buff, he read voraciously about the battles, strategies, and heroism of war. He also loved soccer, basketball, and boxing and was an avid competitor. But John had a dark side, at times verbally abusive and inflexible. His intensity both attracted and frightened people. In retrospect, he would say he was afraid of emotional intimacy. Although many children of the 1960s experimented with drugs, John used them to excess, escaping the emotional pain he was trying to cope with. His controlling nature, along with prolonged periods of well-hidden drug and alcohol abuse, ultimately contributed to the dissolution of his marriage and to the periodic alienation of his two sons. He tried his best to love and accept but too often found himself frustrated, angry, and alone.

John loved coaching soccer. Here his strengths and weaknesses as a person achieved full expression. He was enthusiastic and expressive, driving his players, including his younger son, Josh, to achieve levels of performance well beyond the physical abilities associated with their age. His teams were aggressive and well coordinated, motivated in part by John's exuberance but in part by fear of the excesses of his critical side. He was unrestrained in his praise of outstanding effort, but on occasion he would single out a player who had made an error and publicly chastise him. Josh achieved excellence as a player under his father's intense training, but his need for independence ultimately drove him away from soccer. Josh would later return to play in his senior year, on his own terms, under a different coach. John eagerly anticipated watching Josh play as a spectator, but unfortunately he did not survive long enough to do that.

John knew he was inadvertently alienating his sons, but somehow he just couldn't stop. This pattern did not come out of a vacuum. John's father was a bright, hard-working, progressive thinker who was also emotionally distant, angry, and alcoholic. Nothing John had done as a child had ever been good enough. He thought of himself as lazy and inadequate even at the peak of his career as a journalist. About his mother John said very little other than that she was "crazy," dominating the family with her own emotional needs. Although he had not been physically abused, the scars of his harsh childhood followed John wherever he went. "I never felt I deserved to live," he would say. The tragedy of repeating aspects of his own harsh upbringing with his own children was not lost on John. In spite of his efforts to change, John felt that his children's emotional balance came primarily from their mother.

In an effort to make more sense out of his life and to be a better father, John became involved in both psychotherapy and Zen Buddhism.
In psychotherapy John learned about the present-day effects of his emotional deprivation as a child and explored his fear of intimacy. Beneath
his rage lay a deep depression that he had been trying to dull with alcohol and drugs for years. Through the practice of Zen Buddhism John
learned to live more in the here and now, to stop running from one task
to the next in a futile effort to find meaning and satisfaction.

John was periodically preoccupied by his existential suffering. He
contemplated suicide many times when his isolation and despair felt
overwhelming. He had seen his mother die painfully of ovarian cancer
and was determined not to die by a slow, agonizing process himself.
When John's time came, he would simply "check out," probably by his
own hand. When searching for a reason to keep living, John would
always come back to his two children, whom he loved and of whom he
was prouder than he was of anything else in his life. In his Zen studies
John learned that one's state of mind at death could determine what
might happen in one's next life. He hoped to die in physical comfort
and spiritual peace, surrounded by friends and family. John realized that
to reach that point he had a long way to go. This growth and learning
would not be achieved by working harder according to old patterns,
but rather by initiating a more inward journey that was unfamiliar
to him.

This transformation had already begun when I first met John in the
early 1980s. He came to me with fever, sore throat, swollen glands, and
extreme fatigue that turned out to be infectious mononucleosis. His
liver had been affected, and he was forced to reduce his heavy work
schedule and stop drinking. He initially improved but then began to
feel even more exhausted, sleeping twelve hours a day and awakening
more tired than when he had gone to bed. He felt discouraged, empty,
and completely unmotivated. He withdrew from his family and work.
Depleted by the infection with mononucleosis and then deprived of
the distractions of work and alcohol, John experienced first anger and
then a deep depression. To try to find his way out, he became more in-

tensively involved in psychotherapy. It took him nine months to find his stride. He was not cured of the habits it had taken a lifetime to develop, but he now developed new tools to help him cope and find more fulfillment.

I did not see John again for five years. He returned in 1988 for a complete physical exam, and we reviewed his intervening health and personal history. He saw the infection with mononucleosis as a blessing, forcing him to struggle at a deeper level with the demons that had controlled his life. John was still using drugs and alcohol, but in more moderation. He had left his job in broadcasting to work as a technical writer for a newly formed electronics firm. He had also become the primary caretaker of his two sons, Daniel and Josh. He found common ground with Daniel through books, history, and politics and with Josh in their mutual love of soccer. Although he still had trouble containing his perfectionistic, critical side, John now had achieved enough self-awareness to try to balance it with praise and support. Daniel had received the brunt of John's anger and control when he was a young child. John desperately hoped that they could reconcile their differences, but he knew from his own childhood that such matters cannot be forced. John and his ex-wife, Ellen, continued to scrimmage periodically over financial matters, but they co-parented with reasonable cooperation during these years. His life seemed to be slowly moving in a healthier direction.

I next saw John about one year later. He was feeling lightheaded and slightly dizzy. Josh had beaten him in basketball for the first time, and he was worried about his declining physical abilities. The company he had been working for had closed, and he was unemployed. John was tired, sleeping poorly, unable to concentrate, and extremely depressed. He was waking up in the very early morning, his mind spinning with his unresolved problems. He had no suicidal plans but was isolating himself and thinking of death as an escape from the disaster he was living. I started John on an antidepressant and referred him back to his psychotherapist. His physical examination was normal except for a subtle change in his coordination that was not clear enough to pursue at that time. I advised John to call if his depression or his trouble with co-ordination got worse. We would meet again in several weeks, after he had visited with his therapist several times.

Two weeks later John was admitted to our intensive care unit after experiencing a seizure. He had initially felt better after our last visit. On the morning of his hospitalization, however, he had awakened frightfully ill, vomiting repeatedly and having difficulty walking. He was coherent at first but then became very confused while driving with his son to a soccer game. Josh, then twelve years old, helped him stay on the road. They were found by the police thirty miles out of town, far from their destination. In the hospital John had a series of grand mal seizures and became somnolent and confused. A CT scan showed a mass deep in the center of his brain, most likely an inoperable brain tumor. Pressure from the mass was pushing the remaining brain tissue downward into a fixed space that could not accommodate it. If this herniation of his brain could not be controlled, John would rapidly die.

John's sons, his ex-wife, Ellen, his brother and sister-in-law, and a friend all came to the hospital. I met with them in an urgent, anxiety-filled meeting. John was coming in and out of consciousness, so he could not participate in the initial discussion. His clinical situation was deteriorating, and it was necessary to make decisions rapidly.

"There is a mass deep in John's brain that is pushing down and compressing on the rest of his brain. We are giving medicines to suppress seizures and to limit the amount of swelling around the mass."

"What do you think is causing it?"

"We are not sure, but most likely it is some kind of a growth in the brain."

"Is it treatable?"

How was I to answer this question? Surgery was out of the question, given its location. Radiation might alleviate symptoms for the short term, but it appeared to be a highly lethal brain cancer. Besides, he might not survive the night if his brain kept herniating. They needed to hear the truth but also to maintain some hope. "The treatment is difficult. Surgery is impossible because the lesion is too close to vital structures. We will give John some medication now to limit the swelling and then do a biopsy as soon as possible to see exactly what we are dealing with. There is a new procedure enabling us to do the procedure under CT scan guidance to minimize any further damage to John's brain. Most likely this will be followed by radiation. We are still in a somewhat dangerous situation until the swelling and pressure are controlled."

Terrified and numbed, they had heard enough. I met with John alone. Now more coherent, he wanted to know what was going on. I told him a simple version of the truth, which made him feel frightened and out of control. He was not ready to die—so much unfinished and unsaid.

In the next room, his family was in shock, trying to understand how such a devastating illness could have come on with so little warning. Ellen wondered how much she should be involved, given their divorce and continuing struggles, but she felt she must stay out of loyalty to both John and their children. She wondered privately how John could continue to influence her life so powerfully even as she had successfully struggled to build an independent life for herself. Josh and Dan were trying to be strong but also felt dominated once again by the force of their father's experience. John's brother, David, who probably had the least ambivalent relationship with John, took the lead as John's advocate and support.

The neurosurgeon was enthusiastic about the ability of a new piece of advanced medical technology to do the biopsy with previously unknown precision. In the past, biopsies of tumors in this location had been prohibitively dangerous, often missing the mark and hitting other vital structures. Now the answer could be found without adding to John's already substantial problems. The excitement was limited to the procedure, for both the neurologist and the neurosurgeon were pessimistic about the ultimate outcome. Perhaps John would get a few months if he was lucky, depending on the aggressiveness of the cancer and its responsiveness to radiation therapy. This location in the brain does not tolerate a lot of growth. The biopsy was scheduled for as soon as all the needed technicians and equipment could be organized. We were steeling ourselves for the outcome.

The news from the operating room was ecstatic! We were dealing with *hemophilus aprophilus,* a relatively rare infectious agent that, despite its aristocratic-sounding name, was highly amenable to treatment with common antibiotics! Treatment was started immediately and everyone shared in the joy. Another victory for advanced medical technology! If we could nurse him through six weeks of intravenous antibiotics and avoid complications, what we had thought was a fatal brain cancer would be completely curable. Yet John was not out of the woods. Because of the location of the lesion, a small amount of swelling could still be lethal. But with close monitoring and luck, he should have a full recovery. We had to use the same new technology to drain the lesion a second time, but otherwise John's subsequent recovery went without a major hitch. He had dodged another bullet. With some rehabilitation and hard work, he would again be playing soccer, writing, and living an unrestricted life. We never found an underlying source of infection, and his markers of immune function were all normal. John was still very alive, but it seemed he now had two strikes against him.

John learned a lot from his brush with death. The following is excerpted from an article he wrote that was printed in the *Rochester Democrat and Chronicle:*

> . . . a man who never believed in miracles was presented with several in a matter of weeks, and a second chance at seeing his children grow up.
>
> . . . a man highly skeptical of the medical profession and medical technology was saved by the very newest technology and the brilliance of the neurosurgeon and other doctors.
>
> . . . a man who considered himself a self-sustaining loner survived the most serious crisis of his life through the love and support of his relatives and dozens of friends, and the patient, compassionate care of the . . . nursing staff.
>
> My cynical outlook as well as my brain took a beating last summer.

Reflecting on John's illness, I was once again humbled by medicine's uncertainty and complexity. In retrospect, the slight incoordination I had detected several weeks before his hospitalization had been an early sign of his infection, yet I had chosen not to pursue it because of the pressing nature of his depression. I struggle regularly about whether to use advanced medical technology to study each of my patients' aches or pains. With overtesting, patients become more anxious about their health and more dependent on medical technology than they should be. With undertesting, problems may go undetected while they are still treatable. The challenge is to be alert to what is outside the ordinary and to tolerate those symptoms that are likely to resolve on their own. A small number of these latter symptoms will turn out to be the beginnings of serious illness, so some delay in diagnosis is the price paid for not overtesting and overtreating. When the delay proves potentially dangerous to patients, as was the case with John's infection, it reminds me just how high the stakes sometimes are. Had John not survived, my second-guessing would have been even more painful and sobering.

John made a serious effort to rehabilitate himself both physically and emotionally after his discharge from the hospital. His brain gradually returned to normal, and he was eventually able to play basketball and coach soccer. The fine motor skill needed for playing the guitar was the last to return through his diligent practice. During his illness John grew closer to Ellen. He also made several new friendships that allowed deeper sharing of emotions than he had experienced in the past. The harsh, controlling aspect of John's personality had begun to recede. Illness can be a transforming experience, and John hoped that the next phase of his life would be more enlightened and fulfilling.

John now understood more about the depression that was underneath his anger. He recognized the contribution of his harsh childhood, but he also learned that depression can stem in part from biological problems with neurotransmitters. This revelation helped alleviate some of his guilt about how he had conducted his life, and it opened the door to restarting antidepressant medication, to which he responded very well. He began to feel better than he had at the peak of his broad-casting career, looking inward as well as outward for satisfaction and meaning.

About six months after completing his recovery John found the "perfect job." He was hired as the public affairs officer for the city school district, reporting directly to the district commissioner. It was a creative job that would allow him to use his skills in public relations, research, writing, and project development. He would be a public spokesperson for the district and would report directly to the head of the school system. His boss was innovative and willing to give John considerable independence in carrying out his responsibilities. John had never felt more fulfilled and satisfied.

Unfortunately, John's boss left abruptly two months later to take a job in another city. John's subsequent supervisor had a highly restrictive management style. John chaffed under this kind of control and began feeling angry and rebellious. He increased his drug and alcohol intake and retreated from family and friends. Three months after the transition in leadership, budget cuts in the city school district led to the termination of John's position. John responded viscerally to being unemployed. He frantically looked for work, initially in Rochester, then all over the East Coast. He would be willing to accept a job in public relations, consulting, or advertising. Each night he created a new curriculum vitae to fit his latest idea of what he was going to do.

After two weeks of frantic activity the bottom fell out. "I stopped having a future vision for myself. I could not visualize myself doing anything." The spark of creative energy that had driven him in the past had fizzled, and it seemed impossible to rekindle. His job search became aimless and laconic, and he passively lived off his savings. He dulled the pain, as he had so often in the past, with drugs and alcohol. He thought about suicide but didn't have the energy to take even that seriously. In retrospect, John recognized that he was more depressed than he had ever been in his life, but he was too withdrawn to seek help.

Several months later John began to feel "funny." In addition to having the familiar empty feeling that accompanied depression, he began to sweat excessively at night. One day he felt a pain on the left side of his abdomen. When he examined himself, he noticed a firm, slightly tender area that he had never felt before. Consulting *Gray's Anatomy,* he decided that this was probably his spleen. He knew he was again in medical trouble. Perhaps his self-destructive ways were once more catching up with him.

I was out of town when John came to the office. One of my partners found a hugely enlarged, tender spleen. His liver was also slightly swollen, as were many of his lymph glands. When John asked the covering doctor what he thought was going on, the answer was "possibly a lymphoma" (a cancer of the lymph cells). John couldn't recall the exact name or the conversation, but he knew that the "oma" was not a good sign. His first thought was how he had abused his body over thirty years and that this third illness confirmed that his "immune system was shot." He had read the popular literature about immune vulnerability in settings of loss and grief, and he attributed his current problem to his job loss and his subsequent hopelessness and drug use over the summer. His immediate impulse was to give up and not fight the illness at all. He would hang around as long as he felt okay and then somehow "check out" when his suffering began to increase. He had no interest in living through a long, harsh illness that would end only in his death. He was willing to go through a medical workup to find out exactly what was going on and what the treatment options looked like. Still, in the deepest recesses of his mind he felt a glimmer of hope. He had been lucky twice; perhaps it could happen again.

John's total blood count was normal, but the white blood cells showed atypical, immature lymphocytes. The CT scan of his abdomen confirmed a massively enlarged spleen and multiple enlarged lymph nodes. The only way to make an exact diagnosis was to surgically sample one of these lymph nodes and look at it through a microscope. The clinical picture strongly suggested a lymphoma, but the prognosis and treatment options largely depend on determining the exact cell type. A lymph node in his groin was biopsied in an outpatient procedure. The answer would come within three days. John was uncharacteristically passive during this process, demonstrating relatively little curiosity and making no clear decision about whether he was willing to undertake a medical fight.

His diagnosis was a diffuse, poorly differentiated malignant lymphoma with small cleaved cells, an aggressive, rapidly growing cancer. There is good news and bad news attached to such malignancies. The good news is that the cells are rapidly reproducing themselves, making them very susceptible to chemotherapy. Despite how aggressive the cells appear, these lymphomas are completely curable about 50 percent of the time, provided one completes an intensive course of chemotherapy. The bad news is that the cancer is highly lethal if one doesn't respond to chemotherapy, which also occurs about 50 percent of the time. Without any treatment, death is virtually certain within weeks to months.

John was not sure what to do. He didn't believe the cancer specialists were giving him an honest portrayal of the odds. Because of his pessimistic state of mind and his view that his immune defenses were depleted, he thought his odds of responding to chemotherapy would be considerably less than the 50 percent cited. He had trouble considering chemotherapy when he was already feeling emotionally and physically drained. Unable to activate the fighter within him, he berated himself for the many years of self-destructive behavior as well as the things he had not done for his sons. If these were to be his last months, he did not want to spend them in a hospital being filled with toxic chemicals that would aggravate rather than relieve his suffering.

When I returned, I was saddened to discover that John had contracted yet another serious illness, and I felt somewhat guilty that I had not been there during the diagnostic process. John was well aware that I wrote about end-of-life suffering and that I was, in his words, "not adverse to surrendering when the time comes." He believed he would get an honest opinion from me about whether it was worthwhile for him to proceed. I made it very clear to John that a medical fight using chemotherapy would be worthwhile given his particular cancer and his otherwise healthy condition. With treatment, half of the afflicted patients achieve long-term cure and do not need subsequent treatment. Death was certain without chemotherapy. The fact that the cancer had already spread widely in his body did not change the prognosis.

John later recalled our interview. "I'll never forget what you said to me. You said, 'This is a treatable cancer and you *must* do chemotherapy.' Those were your words. You said, 'You *must* do it.' . . . Having known what you had been through with your other patient, and that you are not adverse to surrendering when the time comes, what you said to me had a tremendous influence." Although I strongly encouraged John to undergo treatment and would have tried to persuade him further if he had chosen not to, the final decision was his to make. He would have to accept the consequences of a decision for treatment, or nontreatment. There was no simple path nor one without considerable risk. Nonetheless, given his good odds of responding to treatment, I thought that it was much too early to opt for no treatment and to make the transition to a palliative approach. Fortunately, John agreed with me.

Part of our discussion about undertaking chemotherapy was an exploration of how John could rediscover the will to live. His entire family was concerned about his discouragement, and each member reached out to him in some way. His isolation and despair had to be explored in order to help him discover a reason to keep going. John's search for hope always led back to his sons. He knew that he had been less than an ideal father, but he hoped to reconnect with them and to participate in their lives in a more meaningful way. Thinking that he could perhaps be a better grandfather than he had been a father, he began to see a future for which he would be willing to fight.

John began to battle his disease instead of himself. He worked with our most aggressive oncologist, whom he described as "the type of guy that you want in a foxhole with you . . . a real go-getter . . . there is no quit in him." John found the oncologist's attitude contagious. He started a regimen of chemotherapy with cyclophosphamide, doxorubicin, vincristine, and prednisone, along with an experimental antinausea drug. There would be a total of eight cycles, approximately one per month. He would know where he stood at the end of that period. It would work or not. And if not? "Well, . . . we will cross that bridge when we come to it." He supplemented this chemotherapy with psychotherapy and completely eliminated alcohol, marijuana, and cigarettes. He joined Alcoholics Anonymous and resumed his Zen practice. He began to visualize his white blood cells fighting off the cancer. Being a military buff, John went to war against the cancer. His white cells were "heavily armed assault troops storming the beach and blasting the crap out of those cells." John was fully activated, fighting for his life, using his inner resources to destroy his disease instead of himself.

The initial signs were very positive. His enlarged lymph nodes disappeared, and his spleen was shrinking rapidly in response to the first cycles of chemotherapy. John found the AA philosophy of "one day at a time" to be particularly important, for his long-term future remained uncertain and frightening when he tried to fully contemplate it. He was feeling closer to Dan, Josh, and Ellen than he had when his physical health was better. The battle was on, and John appeared to be doing everything in his power to ensure a positive outcome.

The first signs that John's cancer might not be fully responding appeared about two-thirds of the way through treatment. His·spleen, which was now less than half its original size, stopped shrinking, and some of his abdominal lymph nodes remained enlarged. The oncologist began talking about ten treatment cycles rather than eight, and some of the drugs would have to be altered to prevent toxicity to his heart. John started to worry, again blaming himself for the years of abuse and neglect. He worried that these "unhealthy" thoughts and fears would further weaken his immune system. He questioned his own inner resolve, feeling that it was his fault that his body was not responding fully to chemotherapy. Perhaps his character was simply too weak to win this battle.

In hopes that the last vestiges of the lymphoma could be eliminated, John completed two additional cycles of chemotherapy. The disease appeared to be about 95 percent gone, but the remaining 5 percent could make all the difference. Additional chemotherapy was recommended. The odds that more treatment would completely dispose of the residual cancer cells, however, were very small. It was also possible that the spleen and lymph nodes had remained enlarged because of scarring rather than cancer. The only way to know for certain would be to do multiple biopsies and possibly exploratory surgery. Having focused all of his energy on completing the recommended course, John could not contemplate further invasive treatment. He was feeling better, and he decided against going further with a medical fight that now looked much less optimistic. The landmarks that we hoped would be very clear at the end of chemotherapy were very uncertain, but John clearly needed a break.

He planned a move to Florida late that summer. Instead of subjecting himself to another Rochester winter, he hoped to enjoy the sun and play golf. His sons could visit and escape the cold. Although he was determined to go, he was operating more on instinct and impulse than on careful planning. We helped him find an oncologist in Florida to ensure good medical follow-up. If his disease recurred, chemotherapy could be initiated at that time. Since the odds that additional chemotherapy would completely eradicate his remaining cancer were very small, I personally felt that John's decision to stop chemotherapy was reasonable. We all worried that his disease was not completely gone, but for now, at least, John could enjoy himself while he felt well. He was also very unsure about how much intervention and suffering he would be willing to put up with if his cancer recurred. "I am not sure if I will want to fight, or if I would rather simply check out." John's future was uncertain, and he would try to take it "one day at a time."

In addition to the warm winter weather and the opportunity to play golf, John was drawn to Florida to be closer to his father. When John had visited him for several weeks earlier that summer they had had a surprisingly good time together. In therapy John had discovered that his father's upbringing had been filled with even harsher deprivation and abuse than had his own. He began to experience some forgiveness and acceptance of his father and hoped this could grow with more regular contact. His father's health was deteriorating, and John hoped they could make peace while they still had time.

Shortly before John's move his father was hospitalized with an acute abdominal problem. John's brother, David, flew to Florida to provide support and to help with decision making. His father emerged from this illness in a very diminished state. He had to be admitted to a nursing home, where he existed for a few months with very poor quality of life. By the time John arrived in Florida his father was near death. John was able to say, "I love you, and I forgive you," as his father lay in a coma, sedated by a morphine infusion. John gave himself a little credit for being with his father during this final process, although his perfectionistic, critical side dwelled on what hadn't been done and said.

John subsequently enjoyed nearly a year in Florida. He was able to live without working by using his savings and the inheritance he received from his father. He felt well, played golf almost every day, made some new friends, and stayed in contact with his family. John began to explore the possibility of going to graduate school. Although the specifics remained hazy, his future began to take shape. He remained relatively optimistic about his cancer, though he simply tried to focus on living each day to its fullest. He maintained his commitment to being free of drugs and alcohol.

Late that spring John noticed the lymph nodes in his groin began to enlarge, and he started to sweat excessively at night. The scenario was all too familiar. He went to see his doctor in Florida, who recommended a biopsy, which confirmed a return of the lymphoma. Shortly thereafter, more lymph nodes began to grow, and the feeling of fullness from his spleen returned. He decided to return to Rochester to be near his family and to explore the next phase of his illness with the doctors he knew best.

John was unsure how to approach his illness. He was faced with a choice between long-shot, experimental therapy with high-dose chemotherapy followed by bone marrow transplantation and a more palliative approach on a hospice program. His first association was with his father's death, which he considered to have been very undignified. He wanted to avoid futile medical treatment, but he also had no desire to live in a severely diminished state that could end only in his death. Yet

John desperately wanted to see his sons grow up and to be a loving grandparent to the next generation. He hoped to write a book about his experience, though he found the creative expression of his inner experience much more challenging than his former writing as a journalist.

John had a lot to live for, but he found that much of his fight was gone. "It's like those guys in the Pacific in the Second World War. How many beaches can you storm before you just give up. . . . I don't know how much fight is going to be required of me at this point, but somewhere I feel that some of the fight has gone out of me. Maybe I'm finally ready to surrender and turn it over to God." Even if he was going to turn his fate over to God, he still had to make the major decision whether to pursue the path of aggressive medical therapy or to pursue hospice care. Neither choice precluded the possibility of a miracle, but the decision would in large measure determine the quality of the last phase of his life. The odds of his responding to chemotherapy and bone marrow transplantation were very small—less than 5 percent; conversely, there was over a 95 percent chance that he would not respond to this treatment, and he would experience the same substantial side effects of treatment in either case.

Given his concern about end-of life suffering, I was somewhat surprised about the clarity with which John made the decision to continue with aggressive therapy. The passivity and acceptance of hospice held no appeal for him. He preferred an active approach: "I'll go down swinging if I have to." John also wanted the possibility of stopping aggressive treatment and even "checking out" if his suffering became too severe. He was quite clear about his intention to take his own life rather than endure suffering that could not be adequately relieved. I assured him that we would work together to face what had to be faced, but I did not look forward to confronting this prospect with him.

John had considerable difficulty with the initial cycles of chemotherapy. His blood counts fell dangerously low, making him vulnerable to infection and bleeding. He developed intractable hiccoughs; he had violent, jerking spasms day and night for weeks at a time that were unresponsive to suppressive measures short of heavy sedation. His pain was relatively well controlled with medication, but the hiccoughs were omnipresent. In his mind, they were "not the sort of thing you check out over." Although treatment was not going well and the odds of response were becoming vanishingly small, John still wanted to continue.

John's massively enlarged spleen seemed to be sequestering many of his other blood cells, thereby lowering his counts and limiting the amount of chemotherapy he could receive. A decision was made to remove the spleen to alleviate this problem, in the hope that this would allow the rest of his treatment program to proceed. John was enthused by the plan despite its considerable risk given his low blood counts and overall condition. His spleen had been the symbolic center of his illness, and he would be glad to be rid of it and get on with the campaign. We were now in a desperate street fight against an overpowering enemy. The rules and strategies were evolving on a daily basis, depending more on intuition than on experimental data.

John went through the surgery with surprising ease. He had very little pain and almost no bleeding. He was up walking the day after surgery, and plans were being made for discharge in the next day or two. His blood counts looked better than they had in weeks. He would go home briefly before resuming chemotherapy. On his third hospital day he was seen on surgical rounds at 6:00 A.M. He was "feeling great and eager to go home." An hour later John was found dead during a routine check. Efforts to resuscitate him were unsuccessful. His "sudden death" came as a complete shock. He had survived so many arduous battles in a war that seemed far from over, only to be killed by a random event, far removed from combat. His autopsy showed no blood clot to his lungs, no undetected bleeding or infection, and no heart attack. John was probably near death from his advanced cancer, and his heart showed the deleterious effects of chemotherapy. His death at that moment in time, however, remains a mystery.

John described himself as an inveterate loner, yet his funeral was attended by hundreds of people. His intensity and enthusiasm were forceful positive counterweights for his perfectionism and anger. Everyone who attended had a powerful story about how John had both touched and challenged them. My own personal experience caring for John was no exception. He was truly a man of contrast and contradiction.

Commentary

1. *Severe illness threatens the integrity of the person.* One's life can be altered in ways that cannot be imagined or minimized, shattering one's self-concept and disrupting one's usual patterns of interacting. Yet, paradoxically, life-threatening illness can also offer new opportunity for affirmation and growth. John would talk vividly about the disintegration and fear that accompanied his illness. Using his omnipresent military metaphors, he spoke of being the pilot of a fighter jet that was spinning out of control, its rudder irreversibly damaged by the latest assault. Should he eject over enemy territory or take his chances in the cockpit? Yet, becoming sick presented John with opportunities to break out of lifelong patterns of self-destructive behavior and to access a range of emotions that included more than anger and self-criticism. Through his three illnesses, each more severe than the one before, John became more able to experience intimacy with his children, his ex-wife, his father, and his brother. He learned to look within as well as outside himself for answers, and he became more able simply to "be with," rather than trying to change, those he loved.

I am not so romantic or naive as to believe that illness is always good for the soul, but I am sure that often some good is possible. When one must confront illness, disability, and even death, the inherent loss and devastation must be acknowledged while simultaneously searching for opportunities for personal growth. The process cannot be rushed or cut short. Hopelessness and despair may need to be felt and shared before new avenues of hope can be discovered. Nonetheless, the opportunity for new forms of fulfillment in the face of severe illness needs exploration and nurturing. John died from his lymphoma, but he also became much more whole as a person before he died.

2. *The mind-body connection can be a double-edged sword for persons trying to make sense out of severe illness.* The life setting in which one be-

comes ill is often significant. John's lymphoma started in the context of his having lost a job on which he had placed high hopes. He was subsequently plunged into depression and increased drug and alcohol abuse. He viewed his illness as stemming in part from his lifelong self-destructive tendencies. "My body was committing suicide" was how he put it. If he changed these patterns, perhaps his body could win the battle against cancer. John transformed this belief into a plan for taking better care of himself. He worked on his depression and created more intimate, supportive relationships. Instead of fighting against himself, he joined his body in the fight against his illness, using visualization techniques along with better nutrition, exercise, and the avoidance of toxic chemicals. Clearly, John used the mind-body connection to his benefit and evolved as a person during this period.

But where did that leave him when his illness didn't respond fully? When he was being absolutely honest, he would admit that he couldn't completely control all of his self-destructive thoughts and feelings. Was that why his illness recurred? Perhaps if he had been stronger or more disciplined . . . Maybe he wasn't being intimate enough with his family, or perhaps he hadn't unearthed the core conflict that would have unleashed his full healing potential. Perhaps he had bad karma from the sins of a past life. The potential for guilt and for second-guessing oneself when treatment doesn't work can undermine the important changes that have been accomplished. An overly simplistic psychosomatic analysis can sometimes form a wedge between patients and their families when treatment doesn't work. Family members may become disappointed in the person rather than in the disease and hold back their support and acceptance. The mind-body connection is important, but it is only one piece of a complex puzzle that determines why people get sick when they do, and who responds and who does not. Sometimes individuals who continue to do all the wrong things survive in spite of terrible odds, while those with good odds who do all the right things die anyway. It is not fair. It is simply what is.

3. *John needed to continue fighting.* John loved the history and stories of World War II, and he was a fan of boxing, soccer, and basketball.

John fought himself when he didn't have other things to fight. This not only made him an outstanding (though feared) interviewer and a hard-driving coach but also contributed to his difficulties in marriage and as a parent. When he was faced with the possibility of death, this fight allowed John to try aggressive treatment both when the odds were good and when the chances of success were remote. The longer the odds, the more heroic was the battle.

Toward the end of his life John was caught in the paradoxical position in which so many dying patients find themselves. He did not want to suffer unnecessarily, but he equated giving up the fight for life with giving in to passivity and despair. Hospice did not appeal to John, for when he stopped fighting his disease, those considerable energies would likely be turned inward, contributing to rather than alleviating his suffering. John wanted to fight until the battle was clearly lost and then "check out" as painlessly as possible. Whether he would have adapted to a hospice approach at the very end or taken his life to escape the dependency and potential suffering, we will never know. John was spared what for him would have been an agonizing decision. He died on the battlefield, probably as he would have wished.

References

Threat of Severe Illness

Cassell, E. J. Recognizing suffering. *Hastings Center Report,* May–June 1991, 24–31.

Delvecchio-Good, M., B. J. Good, C. Schaffer, and S. E. Lind. American oncology and the discourse on hope. *Culture, Medicine and Psychiatry* 14 (1990): 59–79.

Frankl, V. E. *Man's Search for Meaning.* Rev. ed. New York: Washington Square, 1984.

Limitations of Mind-Body Attributes

Barnlund, D. C. The mystification of meaning: Doctor-patient encounters. *Journal of Medical Education* 51 (1976): 716–25.

Barsky, A. J. The paradox of health. *New England Journal of Medicine* 318 (1988): 414–18.

Cohen-Cole, S. A., and C. P. Friedman. The language problem: Integration of psychosocial variables into medical care. *Psychosomatics* 24 (1983): 54–57, 59–60.

Eisenberg, L. Is health a state of mind? *New England Journal of Medicine* 201 (1979): 1282–83.

———. The physician as interpreter: Ascribing meaning to the illness experience. *Comprehensive Psychiatry* 22 (1981): 239–48.

———. The subjective in medicine. *Perspectives in Biology and Medicine* 27 (1983): 48–61.

Holmes, T. H. Life situations, emotions, and disease. *Psychosomatics* 19 (1978): 747–54.

Klerman, G. L., and J. E. Izen. The effects of bereavement and grief on physical health and general well-being. *Advanced Psychosomatic Medicine* 6 (1977): 63–104.

Kushner, H. S. *When Bad Things Happen to Good People.* New York: Avon, 1981.

Sontag, S. *Illness as Metaphor.* New York: Farrar, Straus & Giroux, 1978.

The Need to Keep Fighting

Cowart, D. S. Confronting death in one's own way. *Pain Forum* 4 (1995): 179–81.

Cummins, R. O. Matters of life and death: Conversations among patients, families, and their physicians. *Journal of General Internal Medicine* 7 (1992): 563–65.

Jackson, D. L., and S. Youngner. Patient autonomy and "death with dignity": Some clinical caveats. *New England Journal of Medicine* 301 (1979): 404–8.

Lo, B. Improving care near the end of life: Why is it so hard? *Journal of the American Medical Association* 274 (1995): 1634–36.

Miller, D. K., R. M. Coe, and T. M. Hyers. Achieving consensus on withdrawing or withholding care for critically ill patients. *Journal of General Internal Medicine* 7 (1992): 475–80.

Chapter 7

"You Promised Me
I Wouldn't Die Like This"

Not all patients become well known to their doctors. For some patients the anonymity is a matter of choice, other times inclination, and still others never have the need or the opportunity to develop a close relationship with a physician. Our health care system is chaotic, competitive, expensive, and not universally available. Intimate, longstanding doctor-patient relationships still exist, but they may be more the exception than the rule. Nonetheless, journeying through a complex illness together often creates a closeness between patient and physician to which neither the persons nor the system would otherwise be predisposed.

The commitment not to abandon is present even when patients are not well known to their physicians, particularly if the patient reaches a point of personal disintegration from his or her illness. When patients find themselves dying a "bad death," they should be able to count on medical professionals to be responsive.

Consider Mr. Kline, an eighty-year-old widower in whom cancer of the lung had already spread to his bones when it was initially detected.[1] I did not know him well, having seen him only twice in five years for routine physical exams. Retired from a successful career as a stockbroker, he was a robust man who had always enjoyed good health. He had given most of his energy to his work, though he had always

1. A shorter version of this chapter, written by myself and R. V. Brody, was published as "You promised me I wouldn't die like this!" A bad death as a medical emergency, in *Archives of Internal Medicine* 155 (1995): 1250–54.

found time to play golf and travel. Life seemed to come easily to Mr. Kline. He had a "matter of fact" style; in approaching most complex problems he sought quick, short-term solutions and then moved on to the next challenge.

His wife had done the majority of the child rearing for their son and daughter. Mr. Kline would be present for big events; he was appreciative of his children's achievements but was rather distant from their day-to-day lives. His daughter became a social worker, and his son a schoolteacher; both had married and raised a family. Although they were both sensitive, successful, caring people, Mr. Kline secretly had hoped they might embark on more remunerative careers.

Mr. Kline's wife had held the family together throughout their married life. When the children were on their own, she arranged for annual family reunions and regularly visited with the grandchildren. After her death ten years earlier, Mr. Kline had constructed an active life for himself revolving around his golf club, traveling to visit old friends, and investing his savings in the stock market. He had adjusted to being a widower with outward ease and seemed to need little suport. Without his wife to organize and serve as intermediary, his contacts with his children and grandchildren became increasingly sporadic and uncomfortable. They did not seem to have much in common.

Mr. Kline had never smoked, nor had he had any occupational exposures that would put him at risk for lung cancer. He came to see me because he was losing weight and had a cough that wouldn't quit. He accepted the diagnosis of metastatic lung cancer with relative equanimity. He had expected it. After consulting with one of our medical oncologists, Mr. Kline chose experimental chemotherapy despite its relatively poor track record for his cancer (adenocarcinoma). In making this decision, he described himself as a "battler" who wanted to wage an aggressive fight even if the odds were poor.

Mr. Kline tolerated chemotherapy well and continued to play golf and maintain his social life. Even though he was not cured of his cancer, he responded sufficiently well to remain fully functional for twelve months. Since he was receiving monthly chemotherapy and being followed carefully by the cancer specialists, I did not see him at all. I would be available if questions arose, if the treatment stopped working, or if he had a desire to talk about his illness.

When I next saw Mr. Kline, he had developed severe pain in his neck. X-rays confirmed the recurrence of cancer in the bones of his cervical spine, and we arranged palliative radiation, which provided temporary relief. He understood that his disease was worsening and that further aggressive therapy would be futile, so he agreed to a referral to a hospice program. Having witnessed his wife's death from cancer ten years earlier, he had some specific fears about dying about which he was quite articulate. It was the first intimate detail of his life that he shared with me. In his view, his wife had died a "bad death." She had suffered from uncontrolled pain toward the end, and for her last few weeks she had been "out of her mind" from the sedating effects of analgesic medications. He would much rather die by his own hand than endure something that degrading. Both his hospice nurse and I promised him that "he wouldn't die alone and he wouldn't die in pain." We specifically reinforced our willingness to give him as much pain medicine as he would need.

To qualify for hospice, Mr. Kline had to identify a primary caregiver. This is usually a family member or friend who is willing to stay with the patient, oversee his or her care, and provide hands-on care if necessary. Because his relationship with both of his children had sometimes been strained, Mr. Kline was surprised and appreciative that his daughter was willing to take on this role. Her children were grown and she was not working. She would be able to visit him daily and to stay overnight if the need arose. His son also offered to help, although he was somewhat more reticent and less available because of his ongoing teaching responsibilities. Perhaps Mr. Kline could get to know his children better and make amends for what he had not given them as a father before he died. He had no desire to live a dependent, debilitated life, but he would "hang in there" for a while. Perhaps some good could come out of it.

Mr. Kline's initial three months in hospice included many of the elements of a "good death." Although he had increasing pain in his neck and lower back that included neuropathic components (shocklike, lancinating, electric pains emanating from damaged nerves), we achieved reasonably good control with a combination of oral morphine, which he took around the clock, and antidepressant medication, which seemed to help both his mood and his neuropathic pain. He had regular home visits by the hospice nurses and occasional visits by me as his primary care physician to assess and adjust the regimen. Mr. Kline focused almost exclusively on biomedical issues during our conversations, but he began to have long, meaningful talks with his children. They developed a better understanding of one another and consequently a closer relationship than they had ever had before. As the disease progressed and he became weaker, Mr. Kline accepted his impending death. He had made peace with his children and believed that he would be joining his wife in the afterlife.

During the fourth month of hospice care Mr. Kline's pain in his neck and chest increased dramatically. He got little relief from daily increases in his round-the-clock doses of morphine, and adjustments in adjuvant pain relievers including antidepressants, antiseizure medications, and steroids were not helpful. Unable to sleep, eat, or move without severe pain, he began to visualize himself dying much as his wife had. I made a home visit with his primary hospice nurse to decide what could be done to help. Feeling desperate and out of control, he cried out to us: "You promised me I wouldn't die like this!" He had accomplished what he had hoped for in making better contact with his children. He was no longer afraid of death; indeed he actually preferred it to the condition in which he now found himself. His children were also adamant that something had to be done; sitting at his bedside witnessing the disintegration of this very proud man was intolerable.

After discussing the situation, Mr. Kline, his family, his hospice nurse, and I agreed that he would be best served by a brief admission to the hospital to bring his pain under control. There we could adjust his medicines much more rapidly and aggressively than we could at home. In the hospital he literally begged for help to escape the pain that had enveloped his life. He repeatedly chided himself for not having "taken care of this at home while I still could." We gave him morphine intravenously, rapidly adjusting the dosage upward. Specialists in pain management and palliative care were consulted, and a wide range of additional possibilities was explored, including nerve blocks and neurosurgical procedures. Mr. Kline had already received maximal doses of radiation therapy to the painful areas, and he was adamant that he wanted no more surgery or invasive procedures. He would welcome the sedation that might come from rapidly increasing doses of morphine. We increased the morphine infusion every thirty minutes and gave him bolus doses in between. His pain was well controlled within twelve hours.

Unfortunately, in addition to becoming somnolent, Mr. Kline became paranoid and began to hallucinate. He believed the nurses and his children were his jailers and attackers. He was unable to feel safe despite constant reassurance that he was among friends and loved ones. When the dosage of morphine was lowered to where his mental state was more lucid, the severe pain returned. Changing opioids did not resolve the dilemma. Attempts to mitigate his agitation with benzodiazepines and phenothiazines (minor and major tranquilizers) were unsuccessful. In spite of our best efforts, Mr. Kline was dying a "bad death," feeling totally unsafe and out of control. To add insult to injury, he was also too confused to help with subsequent decision making.

His daughter had previously been named as his health care proxy. Since she was a retired social worker, she knew her responsibilities as a patient advocate. She also saw the caring, commitment, and connection she and her brother had experienced with their father for the first time being undermined with each moment he lingered in this condition.

"We have got to do something! We promised Dad that we would not allow this to happen to him, and yet exactly what he had feared is happening," his daughter lamented. So far we were all on the same side of the fence, but it was clear that Mr. Kline's children were counting on me not to passively let nature take its course. At this moment nature was being far too cruel to Mr. Kline.

"We have a rather delicate situation," I responded. "We have brought your father's pain under control, but in doing so he has become delirious. When we cut down on the pain relievers, his mind gets clearer, but his pain returns. When we increase the medicine further, he gets even more confused." I wanted to be sure we had a common understanding of the clinical situation.

"We can't just leave him in this state. Do we have any options?" his son asked.

"There are some rather radical approaches. We can't keep turning up the opioids, because he is no longer in pain, and besides, they only make him more agitated. We can, however, heavily sedate him using an intravenous infusion of barbiturates to relieve his hallucinations. Once we do this, he will be unconscious, unable to respond and unable to eat or drink. He will be under the equivalent of general anesthesia. But he also will be free of the terror he is now experiencing." Although I had read about this possibility, I had never carried it out. Given current legal restrictions about more direct methods of physician-assisted death, it appeared to be our only option for helping Mr. Kline. It seemed awfully close to euthanasia, but theoretically it was within the confines of the "double effect" as long as our intent was to relieve suffering and not to ease death. To use this treatment, we would need a clear consensus between the patient, his family, and the medical personnel.

"Is this our best choice?" asked his children, looking for guidance.

"It is not ideal, but it is probably the only way to guarantee immediate relief of his suffering. He is near death no matter what we do, and it seems senseless to allow this to continue if we can provide an escape. Our job, however, is to make this decision the way he would want it made if he could speak for himself. I am not asking what we would want for ourselves or what we want for him, but rather what we think he would want for himself. Given our prior conversations, I personally think your father would choose this 'heavy sedation' if he could understand the situation, but I need your input." I was providing them with a recommendation but also reminding us all about substituted judgment: we should try to make the decisions Mr. Kline would make if he could speak for himself.

"He would definitely want an escape—the more rapid and pain-less, the better. He has been very clear from the outset that he would rather be dead than suffer like our mother did. If heavy sedation is his only option, please do it now so this agony doesn't have to continue."

Once Mr. Kline's family and I agreed upon a plan, I then had to en-gage the medical staff currently involved in his care, as well as the hos-pice team, to ensure that they too were comfortable with this intervention. It was especially important that the nurses who would have to administer and monitor the barbiturate infusion understood its intent and its necessity. I presented several articles from the medical literature to document the precedent for such treatment. The hospital nurses and I also had a long history of working together to solve diffi-cult palliative care problems, so trust was not an issue. Many of our nurses had sought guidance from doctors when their patients were dying badly, only to be told that "nothing could be done." The painful reality they faced at Mr. Kline's bedside demanded some kind of ac-tion. Armed with the written information and my personal reassur-ance that barbiturate sedation was within the confines (though on the edges) of currently accepted medical ethics, the nursing staff was ready to assist in the plan. I had a similar conversation with our pharmacist, who helped determine starting doses and concentrations. Fortunately for Mr. Kline, the diverse health care providers worked as a team, learn-ing from and supporting one another through this emergency situa-tion, just as they would for any other patient whose life was at stake.

Mr. Kline was sedated to unconsciousness within three hours using the barbiturate infusion. We began with a relatively low dose but then regularly increased it, using supplemental doses in between, until his hal-lucinations and terror had been alleviated. When the infusion was cut back, the agitation returned. In this sedated state Mr. Kline could not communicate, nor could he eat or drink. He would be "allowed to die" of dehydration and of his underlying disease over the next several days. Our primary intention was to relieve his suffering, not to cause his death, so we were still operating under the confines of the "double effect." Yet, in reality, relieving his suffering and easing death had become one.

Mr. Kline's family was very appreciative of our willingness to provide this unusual solution. Having been intimately involved with their father throughout the last stage of his illness, they understood his wishes. The days before his death, during which he was sedated to unconsciousness, were not unpleasant. Those who had been close to Mr. Kline came by to pay their respects and to say good-bye. Although Mr. Kline could not respond, he appeared peaceful. The stillness in his room, except for his shallow breathing, was in stark contrast to the chaos and disintegration we had all witnessed in the previous days. Yet there was something unsettling about the process. Several family members and friends found it absurd and even cruel to force him to linger in an iatrogenic coma when death was the inevitable outcome. Many commented that we would never put our pets through such a process. Yet every person who had witnessed Mr. Kline's deterioration over the preceding days knew that this was better than allowing him to continue to fall apart.

Mr. Kline died quietly five days later with his daughter and son at his side. His struggle had been minimized for those final days, but it had been a haunting time. Our solution at the end was inadequate; it was simply the best we could do under the circumstances. Those around him, both family and health care providers, worked collaboratively and supported one another. We found solace in fulfilling our commitment not to let him die alone or in pain. This far outweighed the unusual nature of our participation in his death.

Commentary

1. *Not all "bad deaths" can be attributed to the physician's lack of skill and knowledge or to the lack of appropriate resources.* As the story of Mr. Kline's illness illustrates, disease can be diverse and sometimes ruthless. Unforeseen dilemmas emerge every day as we learn new ways to help people live a little longer. Individuals vary considerably in their tolerance for and willingness to accept pain, nausea, dependence, sedation, and the myriad other potential sources of anguish faced by the dying. Fur-

thermore, suffering includes psychological, social, spiritual, and existential dimensions that are often intertwined and less amenable to simple interventions than the more physical aspects. In the Netherlands, where euthanasia is openly tolerated, it is frequently sought because of "loss of dignity," "unworthiness of dying," "dependence on others," and/or "tiredness of life." Though pain is a factor in 46 percent of cases, it is the sole factor in only 5 percent. Clearly, the anguish of dying patients at the very end is more complex and multidimensional than is ordinarily acknowledged.

One of the central commitments physicians should make to their dying patients is that their pain will be managed and they will remain as functional and as mentally alert as possible until their death. Although this is not the same as guaranteeing a pain-free death, it is a commitment to treat pain aggressively. We can generally be more reassuring about pain relief than about symptoms such as nausea, vomiting, open wounds, or dyspnea, but even achieving adequate pain relief without unacceptable adverse reactions is occasionally impossible. Very limited empirical data about pain relief in hospice programs suggest effectiveness ranging from 63 to 100 percent, depending in part on whether patients are being asked or physicians are reporting. My experience suggests that pain relief acceptable to the patient can be achieved about 98 percent of the time, which is reassuring unless you are unfortunate enough to be in the unrelieved 2 percent.

One wonders how Mr. Kline's death and pain control would be coded in such an efficacy-of-care study. He had good pain control most of the time, but he had a period before death when the pain was excruciating and, concurrently, his personhood disintegrated. Longitudinal phenomenological descriptions of patients' experiences in hospice programs may help us better understand the complex realities faced by dying patients, their families, and health care providers. Though dying can be a time of enhanced meaning and conflict resolution, it often has very harrowing moments.

2. *The options available to ease the death of patients dying in agony have recently been extended to include barbiturate sedation and discontinuance of*

eating and drinking. All health care providers who care for severely ill and dying patients must become knowledgeable about a patient's right to refuse or discontinue life-sustaining treatment and about the use of high-dose opioids to treat terminal pain and shortness of breath. If we are to include barbiturate sedation and voluntary dehydration as possibilities for patients who are suffering severely, we must educate doctors, nurses, and patients about their acceptability. Unless we are completely clear about their ethical and legal status, many health care providers will be reluctant to offer them.

Barbiturate sedation is justified under the principle of "double effect." The primary intention is to relieve suffering, and the sedated patient is "allowed to die" of the disease, the barbiturates, and/or dehydration since he or she can no longer eat or drink. Death in these extreme circumstances may be *foreseen,* but must not be *intended,* if it is to remain within the confines of "double effect," no matter how extreme and unacceptable the patient's circumstances. Although pain and agitation can usually be relieved by doses of medication that are not sedating and do not contribute to death, occasionally, as with terminal sedation, the contribution is substantial.

The logic used to justify the right to refuse treatment has been used to justify the possibility of discontinuing eating and drinking. Patients who want to die because their life has become intolerable may now have the possibility of starving, or, more accurately, dehydrating, themselves to death. Presumably, the physician would ensure informed consent, including full consideration of palliative alternatives, and then comfort and relieve symptoms as the process unfolds. The physician's role in these deaths would be ethically "passive," and the patient would be "allowed to die" a natural death (not suicide) from dehydration.

The possibilities of barbiturate sedation and terminal voluntary dehydration, if publicized and openly talked about, would reassure many terminally ill patients and others who fear a "bad death." They make concrete our willingness to provide an escape from most adverse circumstances that patients can imagine. They also allow a culturally acceptable response to those relatively few patients who reach a point at which they welcome death as preferable to their present and foreseeable future life. It may not be the method they would choose if all options were available, but at least continued agony would not be enforced. These options would also be of value to those doctors and patients who find great meaning in the current ethical distinction between "active" and "passive" roles in assisting dying and who would find directly assisting death and suicide to be immoral even in the face of irreversible anguish. While severely testing the edges, these methods can be conceptualized within the confines of the "double effect" and the right to refuse treatment. Even if the laws change to permit physicians to more directly assist death, acceptance of such change will occur very slowly. In addition, we will still need the widest range of options in order for actions to be congruent with the values of individual patients and their caregivers.

A patient of mine who had advanced breast cancer was becoming discouraged about a future that potentially held only further disability and dependence. After five years of adjusting to the repeated challenges of her slowly spreading cancer, her specific fear was that she would be deprived of determining when she had had enough and was ready to die. She had read a newspaper account of the death of Dr. David Eddy's mother.[2] Mrs. Eddy, an elderly woman who was ready to die but did not have an imminently terminal condition, chose to completely stop eating and drinking. She was thereby able to ensure her wished-for death without compromising either her family or her physician. My patient found the report strangely liberating. In spite of my reassurance that I would work with her, she was becoming more and more fearful about her future. Her energy improved and her mood lifted with the knowledge that she could make her own choice, without worrying about whether I would be willing to take a major risk on her behalf or would turn down her request because I didn't think she was suffering enough. That the possibility of starving and dehydrating one-

2. See D. M. Eddy, A conversation with my mother, *Journal of the American Medical Association* 272 (1994): 179–81.

self to death could be found so freeing gives one a small sense of just how desperate and powerless many severely ill patients must feel.

3. *The options of barbiturate sedation and terminal voluntary dehydration clearly broaden the range of suffering that can be addressed.* Barbiturate sedation and terminal voluntary dehydration allow incurably ill, tormented patients who are not in severe physical pain and who are not on life support a potential escape. However, many patients would find spending their last days before death sedated to the point of unconsciousness unacceptable and even absurd. Consciousness and interpersonal connection are fundamental to many persons, and lying in a bed sedated, passively dehydrating, may seem humiliating. A central principle in the care of the dying is to individualize care as much as possible. If we are going to ease death, why not do it in a forthright manner consistent with the values of the persons involved?

Furthermore, barbiturate sedation and terminal voluntary dehydration stretch our principles close to the breaking point. Do our intentions with barbiturate sedation stay within the confines of the "double effect"? Is a wished-for death under those circumstances really unintended or even a "bad" outcome? Are the differences between this act and voluntary active euthanasia worth preserving? Should stopping eating and drinking be considered a variation on the right to refuse treatment, or is it a form of suicide? Clearly, such acts cannot be categorically judged without considering the motives, intentions, and circumstances of the actors. Sometimes stopping eating and drinking to seek death should be considered a form of suicide (a patient with clinical depression or anorexia nervosa), and other times it should be considered consistent with "allowing to die" (a competent terminally ill patient in agony who has no other options). Some severely suffering patients would prefer a quick, explicit act to end life rather than a solution that requires them to go through a period of sedation and dehydration before death. Yet even these patients, like Mr. Kline, would usually prefer a sedated death to continued, unrelieved torment.

4. *Bad deaths require a vigorous medical response.* The disintegration experienced at the very end by patients like Mr. Kline should be consid-

ered a medical emergency. Mr. Kline took advantage of experimental chemotherapy to extend his life, but in doing so he also unwittingly accepted the risk that unforeseeable complications might arise in his future. When aggressive treatment stopped working, he made a timely transition to hospice care. He was thereby able to use his final months to connect with his children more meaningfully than he had when he was healthier. The family healing that occurred during this period, however, was severely threatened when his symptoms later became overwhelming and uncontrollable. We fulfilled our commitment to relieve his physical pain, but the result was that he became delirious. He began to literally live a nightmare with no end in sight other than his death. Medical professionals must be empowered and obligated to act in the face of such disintegration. Forcing patients and doctors to let nature take its course under these harsh circumstances, especially after having previously intervened so aggressively and "unnaturally," is morally unacceptable. Our obligation not to abandon requires that we search for and find acceptable solutions.

Stopping life-sustaining therapy and treating terminal pain with increasing doses of opioids provide an adequate escape for most patients. But sometimes, as with Mr. Kline, standard methods either do not work or create unanticipated additional problems. Physicians are then obligated to keep searching for answers that stay within the value structure of both patient and doctor but also resolve the problem. If patients lose the capacity to speak for themselves, we must work with their families to try to intervene as the patients would want us to. Heavy sedation with barbiturates in Mr. Kline's case might seem a bizarre solution at first, but it was better than allowing Mr. Kline to linger in a state of anguish that could end only in his death.

The stakes under these agonizing circumstances are very high. Even though Mr. Kline could no longer speak for himself, his personhood still lay in the balance. During such medical emergencies physicians are sometimes forced to use extraordinary methods. Our patients are counting on us not to be afraid to act on their behalf.

References

Severe Suffering in the Face of Good Palliative Care

Battin, M. P. *The Least Worst Death: Essays in Bioethics on the End of Life.* New York: Oxford University Press, 1994.

Cohen, M. H., A. Johnston-Anderson, S. H. Krasnow, and R. G. Wadleigh. Treatment of intractable dyspnea: Clinical and ethical issues. *Cancer Investigation* 10 (1992): 317–21.

Coyle, N., J. Adelhardt, K. M. Foley, and R. K. Portenoy. Character of terminal illness in the advanced cancer patient: Pain and other symptoms during the last four weeks of life. *Journal of Pain and Symptom Management* 5 (1990): 83–93.

Dobratz, M. C., R. Wade, L. Herbst, and T. Ryndes. Pain efficacy in home hospice patients: A longitudinal study. *Cancer Nursing* 14 (1991): 20–26.

Ingham, J., and R. Portenoy. Symptom assessment. In *Pain and Palliative Care,* ed. N. I. Cherny and K. M. Foley, *Hematology/Oncology Clinics of North America* 10, no. 1 (1966): 21–39.

Kasting, G. A. The nonnecessity of euthanasia. In *Physician-Assisted Death,* ed. J. M. Humber, R. F. Almeder, and G. A. Kasting, 25–43. Totawa, N.J.: Humana, 1994.

Miller, F. G. The good death, virtue, and physician-assisted death: An examination of the hospice way of death. *Cambridge Quarterly of Healthcare Ethics* 4 (1995): 92–97.

Mount, B. M., and P. Hamilton. When palliative care fails to control suffering. *Journal of Palliative Care* 10 (1994): 24–26.

Nelson, J. L. Pain, suffering, and other sources for support for physician-assisted suicide and euthanasia. *Pain Forum* 4 (1995): 182–85.

Ventafridda, V., C. Ripamonti, F. DeConno, M. Tamburini, and B. R. Cassileth. Symptom prevalence and control during cancer patients' last days of life. *Journal of Palliative Care* 6 (1990): 7–11.

Walsh, T. D. Symptom control in patients with advanced cancer. *American Journal of Hospice and Palliative Care* 6 (1992): 32–40.

Barbiturate Sedation

Cherny, N. I., and R. K. Portenoy. Sedation in the management of refractory symptoms: Guidelines for evaluation and treatment. *Journal of Palliative Care* 10 (1994): 31–38.

Cohen, M. H., A. Johnston-Anderson, S. H. Krasnow, and R. G. Wadleigh. Treatment of intractable dyspnea: Clinical and ethical issues. *Cancer Investigation* 10 (1992): 317–21.

Mount, B. M., and P. Hamilton. When palliative care fails to control suffering. *Journal of Palliative Care* 10 (1994): 24–26.

Quill, T. E. "You promised me I wouldn't die like this!" A bad death as a medical emergency. *Archives of Internal Medicine* 155 (1995): 1250–54.

Truog, R. D., C. B. Berde, C. Mitchell, and H. E. Grier. Barbiturates in the care of the terminally ill. *New England Journal of Medicine* 327 (1992): 1678–82.

Terminal Hydration

Bernat, J. L., B. Gert, and R. P. Mogielnicki. Patient refusal of hydration and nutrition: An alternative to physician-assisted suicide or voluntary active euthanasia. *Archives of Internal Medicine* 153 (1993): 2723–27.

Eddy, D. M. A conversation with my mother. *Journal of the American Medical Association* 272 (1994): 179–81.

Fainsinger, R., and E. Bruera. The management of dehydration in terminally ill patients. *Journal of Palliative Care* 10 (1994): 55–59.

McCann, R. M., W. J. Hall, and A. Groth-Juncker. Comfort care for terminally ill patients: The appropriate use of nutrition and hydration. *Journal of the American Medical Association* 272 (1994): 1263–66.

Printz, L. A. Terminal dehydration, a compassionate treatment. *Archives of Internal Medicine* 152 (1992): 697–700.

Chapter 8

Friendship and Hemlock

JANE AND I felt an immediate connection. Although we were "Mrs. Smith" and "Dr. Quill" for the initial ten years of our relationship, our encounters were both medical and personal from the outset. She was a nurse with a strong interest in palliative care even before it became formalized into the hospice movement. In her later years she became a gifted teacher who enjoyed engaging students at all stages of development. She was divorced and had no children. Both of her parents were dead. She lived alone and had a full social life and many good friends. She loved being active and outdoors and was an avid tennis player and golfer. She had just purchased a small country home outside Rochester and planned to spend as much of her summers there as possible.

In her mid-thirties Jane had a near-death experience that transformed her life. She suffered severe brain injury and almost died from a motor vehicle accident. Struggling for her life in the intensive care unit and unable to respond verbally, she hazily recalled receiving last rites. For several days she lived in a twilight between life and death; she later described this transitional state as bright, warm, clear, and tremendously appealing. As she returned to conscious life and had to cope with excruciating headaches, Jane would fondly return to the memories of that peaceful state. Although her spirituality was not formed by an organized religion, she was confident about the existence of a beneficent God. She would welcome life after death rather than fight death off when her time came. She had "embraced the light" and knew that she had nothing to fear.

When we first met I was in still in residency training. My outpatient experience was in a health maintenance organization of which she was a member. She appreciated my willingness to listen and wanted to learn how the relative roles of doctors and nurses would evolve in the next generation. We devoted much of our initial time together figuring out how she could stop smoking. It was an important triumph when she quit, since smoking was especially dangerous given her problems with asthma and high blood pressure. In addition to her medical challenges, we also discussed our common interests in nature, sports, politics, and medicine. I always looked forward to our wide-ranging conversations.

In 1980, after my residency and fellowship, I started my own medical practice. I was pleased to learn that Jane had changed insurance plans so she could remain my patient. Over the past three years she had weathered several severe bronchial infections under my care, and we had formed a strong bond. She appeared to be developing premature emphysema in addition to her asthma. Adding further insult to injury, an inflammatory arthritis began to emerge in the small joints in her hands and feet. It had all the characteristics of rheumatoid arthritis, although the blood serology tests used to confirm the diagnosis remained normal. She was now unable to play golf or tennis as often as she had, but otherwise she remained socially active.

We continued to meet several times each year, usually because of respiratory problems. In order to remain stable, Jane required multiple medications each day—pills for asthma, blood pressure, arthritis, and postmenopausal hot flashes, as well as a variety of inhalers and nasal sprays. In 1982 she scheduled a complete physical exam. Her lungs showed more wheezing and congestion. Formal pulmonary function tests documented another decline in her breathing capacity. A routine mammogram showed abnormal calcifications that a biopsy determined to be from breast cancer. Her medical options were a mastectomy (complete removal of her breast) or a lumpectomy (removal of the affected area only) plus radiation. To my surprise, she chose the more invasive surgery. She had no confidence in radiation in spite of the data showing its effectiveness, and losing her breast was not overly significant to her.

Jane's breathing held up surprisingly well during the surgery, although she hated being in the hospital and depending on others for her care. A preset schedule determined when she was given her medicines, and she had several episodes of wheezing in between the carefully timed doses when she was not able to independently access her inhalers. The fact that "they" rather than she determined when and how she needed to be treated was unnerving, and she was greatly relieved to be released and back in charge of her own life.

Fortunately, her cancer was identified at a very early stage. All of her lymph nodes were clear of tumors, and there were no other signs of distant spreading. She would not need chemotherapy or hormonal therapy. She was likely cured, and preventing a cancer from developing in her other breast was our highest priority. Even though her cancer cells were not very sensitive to estrogen when their receptors were tested, we recommended that she stop hormone replacement therapy. Unfortunately, her hot flashes returned with a vengeance. She had constant sweating, tingling of her skin, and insomnia. Over the next year we tried a series of measures to limit her postmenopausal symptoms and solicited additional ideas from several specialists. Despite our collective efforts, her symptoms were unrelenting. As a last resort, we looked carefully at the tradeoff between the small risk of breast cancer associated with estrogen therapy and the persistent undermining of the quality of her daily life without hormone replacement. To Jane, relief of her symptoms was well worth the risk. I agreed that the decision was hers to make and that the medical risks seemed relatively small given the intractability of her symptoms. Yet if her cancer recurred, or if she developed cancer in her other breast, we would both be subject to second-guessing, since this intervention went against prevailing medical norms. Hot flashes and insomnia may seem trivial compared with cancer when considered from a distance, but for Jane the choice was clear. Since her quality of life was becoming restricted by asthma and arthritis, improving seemingly minor daily discomforts became a high priority.

In 1983 Jane was hospitalized for a lung infection that dangerously compromised her already limited ability to breathe. She required high doses of corticosteroids, and experienced extreme agitation and anxiety as a predictable side effect. She was jumping out of her skin, she couldn't sleep, and she couldn't control her thoughts, which became dominated by a fear of suffocation. Mild tranquilizers did not help. When one feels threatened by suffocation, the call button and the good will of the nurses are vital links between life and death. Most of the staff were responsive, understanding Jane's vulnerability and fear and accepting her need to be in charge of her treatments. A few saw her need to be actively involved as a threat, an invasion of turf that was theirs rather than hers. The hospital began to feel unsafe to Jane, especially at night, when her fears about suffocation and her need to be in control would become accentuated. This intensely independent woman now felt vulnerable as never before.

That winter, while vacationing in Arizona, Jane was again hospitalized with pneumonia, complicated by her asthma. The same fears emerged, but they were more intense and more frightening because she didn't have a physician to advocate on her behalf with the hospital staff. She deteriorated to the point that she needed monitoring in the intensive care unit and was on the verge of requiring a breathing machine. The high-dose steroids needed to treat her asthma again made her anxiety more extreme and her fear inconsolable. When she returned to Rochester, we made another aggressive search for any aspect of her condition that might be reversible. We discovered that she had mild alpha-1-antitrypsin deficiency, a congenital enzyme abnormality that makes one's lungs especially vulnerable to emphysema. Although this discovery made her premature development of severe pulmonary disease more comprehensible, unfortunately it did not open up any new avenues for treatment. We did discover that she was allergic to several molds and pollens, so allergy shots were initiated. She decided to spend subsequent winters in Arizona, avoiding the adverse effects of the cold Rochester winter on her asthma.

Jane managed to avoid the hospital for the next five years, but she was not without several additional medical challenges. Her vision was threatened by a series of retinal tears, requiring close monitoring and repeated laser surgeries. The prednisone needed to control her asthma helped her arthritis, but she developed a "moonlike" face, weight gain, worsening hypertension, and compression fractures of her spine. She needed ten different medications, or more than fifty daily doses, to function. Despite the many compromises, she still enjoyed life. She had good friends both in Arizona and in Rochester, and her social calendar was always full. On good days she could even play nine holes of golf using a cart.

During this relatively stable time in Jane's life I published my article about Diane in the *New England Journal of Medicine*.[1] In response to that article, many people related to me how their lives had been personally touched by end-of-life suffering and how they had felt abandoned by the medical profession. My own patients told me stories they had never shared before about their personal experience with dying family members and friends. Some of their stories were profoundly disturbing. Rather than being frightened by my participation in Diane's death, most found it reassuring. Although they might not choose this option themselves, they now knew that I would not shy away from difficult decision making if they faced a complicated crossroads at the end of their lives. My office hours took on a new intensity.

Jane was one such patient. Although we had discussed our common commitment to palliative care, Jane had never before told me that she had long been a member of the Hemlock Society. She then related the following powerful story, which provides a sobering context for Jane's final chapter.

Bill

Bill was a physically fit, energetic man in his mid-seventies who still worked part-time when he wasn't playing tennis or golf.[2] He lived life

---

1. See T. E. Quill, Death and dignity: A case of individualized decision making," *New England Journal of Medicine* 324 (1991): 691–94.

2. This story was originally published in T. E. Quill, *Death and Dignity: Making Choices and Taking Charge* (New York: W. W. Norton, 1993), 117–20. Copyright Timothy E. Quill; reprinted with permission.

fully and was a joy to be with because of his thoughtfulness, sensitivity, and wit. His first encounter with a serious illness came when he suddenly lost the vision in the center of both of his eyes from a disease called macular degeneration. Legally blind, he was no longer able to read, drive, or enjoy sports that required fine hand-eye coordination. Although he was devastated by this loss, he began to adjust and develop new skills to deal with his deficit.

Several months later Bill was found to have cancer in his throat. Because the cancer had already spread to the lymph glands in his neck, Bill was not a candidate for operative treatment. Instead, he was offered treatment with radiation, which he was told had a good chance of controlling the disease. To take advantage of this chance, he would have to tolerate a sore mouth, difficulty swallowing, and perhaps some trouble hearing in the short term. With little hesitation or questioning, he began radiation treatment.

The reality of the radiation treatment was unfortunately harder than he had imagined. He permanently lost most of his hearing, and he could not swallow solid foods. Though the tumor shrank, the hearing loss and the inability to eat solid foods persisted. He adjusted as well as he could to these severe losses, but his energy and love of life never fully returned.

Over the subsequent eighteen months Bill progressively lost weight. He had constant headaches, and walking short distances left him exhausted. His cancer began to grow rapidly, and it became difficult even to swallow liquids. It had also spread to his sinuses and his brain. He had such large amounts of drainage from his nose that he had to wear a pad under it to keep himself dry. Bill found the draining fluid to be humiliating, a constant outward reminder of his physical degradation. This once active, joyful, very proud man was now legally blind, severely hearing impaired, constantly leaking mucus, and unable even to swallow his own secretions. After two years of progressive loss and misery, it could only get worse.

Jane (my patient) was a retired nurse and a former hospice worker, as well as a member of the Hemlock Society. As a friend of the family with special knowledge and experience, she was called on for advice because of Bill's rapidly deteriorating condition. Bill's wife confided, with tears streaming down her face, that he was now actively thinking about committing suicide. She asked Jane to talk to Bill, and Jane consented. Bill's first words were, "I suppose you're going to try to talk me out of it too." When she replied that she would not, Bill spoke openly of his anguish and helplessness, how he was comforted only by the potential release that would come with death. He dreaded the process of dying much more than death itself, and he could no longer stand the indignity that continuing to live required. He talked at length about his love for his wife and of the unbearable frustration of being a burden for so long.

After several daily visits with Bill and his wife, there was no doubt in Jane's mind that Bill would take his life with or without anyone's approval. He never faltered in his belief that it was his only realistic option. Bill's wife gradually came to accept his decision, though she felt overwhelmed and powerless to help. When they began to discuss methods, Bill brought out a shotgun. They then explored using an overdose of medications as recommended by the Hemlock Society. They discovered that Bill probably had enough potentially lethal medication for the suicide provided he could swallow it all and provided someone would assist with a plastic bag if the overdose were insufficient. (The use of a plastic bag is a backup measure described in the Hemlock Society's literature.) Jane's understanding and compassion for Bill now superseded her concern about her own legal liability if her role in his suicide were discovered. She was committed to being with Bill and his wife until the end.

A plan was made for Bill to take the overdose on his own the next day. Jane would assist with the plastic bag only if necessary. Elaborate plans were made concerning notifying the authorities and what to report. Once Bill was dead, they would remove the bag and call the doctor to report that Bill had been found dead of "natural" causes. Jane went home that night uncertain about what the next day would bring but certain that Bill believed death was his best choice. She left Bill and his wife in a tearful embrace.

When Jane returned the next day, Bill told her that after deliberating all night he had decided not to involve her in his death. He was worried about the legal vulnerability that she and his wife might incur if their assistance in his death were discovered. Despite Jane's protestations that she was willing to take this risk, he was unwilling to change his mind. "I love you too much to risk your future." After a long conversation, Bill excused himself to go to the bathroom. Within minutes there was a loud gunshot. Bill had shot himself through the head. Bill's wife and Jane ran in the direction of the noise, knowing what he had done but not knowing what they would find. They found Bill gruesomely wounded, half-dead and half-alive.

An ambulance and the police arrived and took Bill to the hospital at high speed with sirens wailing. Bill's wife was completely numb, unable to think clearly or speak. Jane felt impotent, enraged, and overwhelmed. They remained behind, not knowing what to do as the ambulance crew whisked Bill away. After Bill was evaluated and resuscitated in the emergency department, it was evident that he was fatally wounded. A physician called the home to inform the family that they might not be able to save him. To Jane's plea, "Please don't try. He's suffered enough," the physician responded, "I'll give him something for his pain and try to keep him comfortable."

Bill died three hours later. His wife will probably never recover or forgive herself. Jane will never forget and is more frightened than ever about the potential of unremitting end-of-life suffering.

It surprised me that Jane had never before shared this experience with me, especially since we had had extensive discussions about the care of the terminally ill. Jane related Bill's story without making explicit her own plans for the future, although I knew that her fear of suffocation was much greater than her fear of dying. She had already experienced extreme shortness of breath, which she hoped never to repeat. I wondered whether Jane's future would lead us to uncharted waters. Although I remained steadfast in my commitment not to abandon my suffering patients in the last phase of their lives, my recent appearance before a grand jury after writing about Diane's story left me sobered and somewhat fearful about my own legal and professional vulnerability.

Jane spent much of that winter in an Arizona hospital. Her breathing deteriorated, and she now required high doses of corticosteroids and constant oxygen to survive. The steroids were associated with all the predictable complications, including worsening hypertension, significant weight gain, edema in her legs, and diabetes mellitus. She lost her voice from the constant coughing, and she became fatigued and short of breath with minimal activity. She came to my office that spring in a wheelchair, oxygen in tow, exhausted by the trip. Her list of medications now numbered fifteen, totaling more than sixty doses each day. They all seemed essential. She had developed pulmonary hypertension, and the right side of her heart was failing. She had to sleep sitting up, the veins in her neck were distended, and fluid was accumulating in her legs. She refused hospitalization ("I'm more afraid of being there than I am of being home"), so we added two more medicines to her growing list and arranged for nursing visits at home. I planned to see her in one week, and she agreed to be hospitalized if her condition worsened.

Two days later, Jane could not catch her breath in the middle of the night. She felt as if she were drowning in her own secretions. She called an ambulance and was rushed to a rural hospital near her home. She was not getting enough oxygen, and she was overloaded with fluid. With constant attention in their intensive care unit, Jane turned the corner without going on a breathing machine. She left the hospital one week later, exhausted and defeated. Walking across her bedroom to the bathroom left her depleted. Her friends and home health aides helped her with meals and with other routine activities, but the independent life she cherished was rapidly disappearing.

I saw Jane later that month. Her skin was battered and bruised and her muscles were weakened from the constant use of corticosteroids. Tired and frustrated, she could see no prospect of improvement. Although she appreciated the help of her friends, she did not like having to depend on them. Her lively mind was trapped in a deteriorating body. She did not want to die, but she also did not want to continue living in such a diminished state. Because she never wanted to go onto a breathing machine but also was terrified of suffocation, I promised that she could be sedated with morphine if her respiratory status ever reached an irretrievable stage.

We completed a do-not-resuscitate (DNR) document for her use in her home as well as in the hospital to ensure that she would not be put on a ventilator. She had already executed a living will, making known her wishes for comfort measures only if she ever became mentally incapacitated. We agreed to try only those measures that might improve her quality of life without putting her through any added suffering. The community health nurse would help organize new respiratory treatments at home and arrange for assistance with housework, shopping, and personal care. We made minor adjustments in her medicines and agreed to meet in one month to see how she was progressing.

Jane was relatively stable over that month. She would probably not survive another infection without the assistance of a ventilator, but it was unclear whether she would rapidly fall off the cliff or continue to die in agonizing pieces. Jane now saw no future to which it would be worthwhile for her to further adapt. She was ready to die. There was no reason to keep going. She could die by stopping all her medicines (patients have the "right to refuse treatment"), but death would come slowly, from asphyxiation. When she began to struggle, we could comfort her with morphine, but Jane knew from her experience as a nurse that these processes do not always go smoothly even in the best of hands.

We then had the following conversation:

"I am not sleeping at all well. I was hoping you would give me some secobarbital to help me sleep better." Jane had a long history of insomnia, and we had tried the gamut of sleeping medicines in the past with little success. I could take her request at face value, give her the medicine, and pretend not to hear her real request. It would be by far the safest thing to do from a legal perspective. Ignorance is bliss. But this was too important a decision to make without a direct conversation. I knew that secobarbital, a barbiturate, was a central ingredient in one of the Hemlock Society's forms of "self-deliverance," and I also knew that Jane was a member. I chose to keep our relationship honest and our conversation out in the open.

"I was afraid that you were going to ask me this." I made her be more explicit about what she was asking. I was not the leader in this conversation but a very reluctant follower.

"I can't stand living this way. This is not living any more. My life has no joy or meaning, and it will only get worse in the future. I can't hold out living on my own much longer, and I have no desire to live as more of an invalid than I already am. Besides, there is no chance that I will get better. I might survive a little longer, but this is not living. I don't want to compromise you in any way, so you should feel free not to provide them."

"I need to know you are sure, and you have considered all the alternatives. I also want to be certain you are not clinically depressed."

Jane laughed. "I am certainly not happy, but I am also not depressed. I have hung on a lot longer than I thought I would, but this summer has been well over the line of what I consider to be tolerable. I am terrified of waiting to suffocate and then, once that starts, not knowing if those around me will have the courage to do what needs to be done. I have seen people dying of suffocation, drowning in their secretions, struggling on and off for days. I have already suffered beyond my limits."

Jane spoke compellingly and accurately about her own physical and existential situation. She had no good choices. I could guarantee her that I would not be afraid to give her enough medicine once she started to suffocate, but I was not available twenty-four hours a day and she lived a considerable distance outside of Rochester. Even if I were available, there would be considerable uncertainty about how the process would go. How much morphine could I give her at the outset and still stay within the confines of the "double effect"? If I gave too much, might that not be considered euthanasia? If I gave too little, might she not suffer unnecessarily?

Besides, she would counter, I would rather die in my own home, surrounded by friends, at a time of my choosing. I cannot stand the way I am living right now, waiting for the end.

"Do you have a plan?" I asked.

"Not exactly," she responded. "The pills will be my security blanket for now. I may even try them for sleep since you know how poorly I sleep."

Jane put the ambiguity back into her request largely for my benefit. If I prescribed the secobarbital with the intent that she use it for sleep, I was on safe legal ground. If I prescribed it in order to give her the security that there could be an out but without the intention that she take it, then I would be in a legally gray zone. If I gave her medicine that I knew she planned to take in an overdose, then my legal vulnerability would be greater, but only if the entire process were uncovered. No wonder these transactions are often veiled and inexplicit.

Yet this was a life-and-death decision. There was no room for confounding it with double meanings and ambiguous statements.

"Jane, I will provide you with the medication, though I am not overly comfortable with it. My discomfort is partly for you since I want to be sure you have explored all the alternatives and are 100 percent certain. There is no turning back on this decision, so I want to meet with you several times to ensure that you still feel completely clear. If you need hospitalization in the interim, I promise that if you become extremely short of breath and are ready to die, I will give you enough morphine so that you won't linger and won't have to beg in any way to get more. You will be in the driver's seat, and I will support your decisions. For now I will give you an average amount of the seconal that would be used for sleep but not for overdose."

Jane brightened considerably after our conversation. She left feeling more optimistic and in control than she had in years. She came back for two follow-up visits, at which she remained steadfast in her desire to escape in a way of her choosing. She continued to take her sixteen regular medications religiously. She began saying good-bye to her friends, letting them know that she did not expect to last much longer. Her friends were surprised about how peaceful she seemed in light of how poorly the last eighteen months had gone. In each of the two subsequent visits Jane told me with a twinkle in her eye that the secobarbital was helping her sleep better and then requested a refill. I was as sure that she was not lying as I was that she was not taking them. After her third visit, I knew she would have accumulated enough medicine to successfully overdose if she had been stockpiling. I asked if she had a plan, and she again responded, "Not exactly." Given my recent legal difficulties, I didn't feel that I could be physically present with her at the very end. However, I needed to be sure that she would not be alone. No one should have to die alone. Jane reassured me that she had good friends who would support her to the end. We scheduled a follow-up appointment, knowing that she probably would not be there.

"Perhaps you will change your mind," I offered.

"Perhaps, but I doubt it," Jane responded. We said good-bye with a hug, tears in our eyes. We probably would not see one another again.

I felt unnerved by these exchanges with Jane. On the one hand, I fully acknowledged that her options all seemed inadequate. She was hovering on the edge of dying from severe cardiopulmonary problems that would only get worse with time. Having suffered beyond her capacity to cope, she had made a decision consistent with her longstanding values. She simply had taken the "least worst" option. On the other hand, our transaction felt very incomplete. I would have liked to get a second opinion but could not do so without putting Jane, the consultant, and myself in legal jeopardy. I had to let her go without full knowledge about her plan and without being able to support her through this final process. Would she die alone, or be terrified at the end? Would she agonize about the final act but feel that she must refrain from calling me in order to protect me from legal problems? What if things went wrong and she couldn't swallow the pills? What if the pills didn't work? What would my legal vulnerability be if the act were discovered? Would it be handled quietly by the medical examiner, or would it become another media circus? I was torn between my duty to respond to Jane and my need to protect myself. I felt as if I were helping her and abandoning her in the same moment.

I was left with more questions than answers and many unresolved feelings. My experience with Jane reinforced my belief that a more open process would have to be better for both patients and doctors than one shrouded in secrecy and ambiguity. These decisions are hard enough without their having to be made underground.

Jane did not come in for her next appointment. I did not call her. I hoped that no news was good news. There was no call from the medical examiner. I hoped she had died in peace and comfort, with her personhood in tact. I hoped she was in a better place, finally finding some peace. But there were too many loose ends for such a profound experience.

About six months later Carol, a long-term patient of mine who had originally been referred by Jane, made an appointment for an acute problem. Out of the blue she said, "I want to thank you for helping Jane." My stomach tightened and my sensors went onto full alert. I took a deep breath and asked, "What happened?" She then completed Jane's story for me.

Jane made up her mind not to return to Arizona. Carol and Jane were intimate friends, having supported one another through several difficult life transitions in the past. Having witnessed Jane's recent decline and knowing her philosophy about the end of life, Carol was not surprised by Jane's plan. They both had strong faith in the existence of an afterlife, though the steps of getting from here to there seemed uncertain and treacherous. Nonetheless, Carol promised to provide Jane with support and assistance. She would be her partner and friend no matter what happened.

Another mutual friend, Sarah, also vowed to stay with Jane. Sarah kept hoping she could convince Jane to change her mind. If only she tried a little harder and gave a little more, perhaps Jane would keep going. Sarah was more uncertain about death and skeptical about the existence of an afterlife. Without this comforting vision, the prospect of assisting Jane during her last hours was especially daunting. Nonetheless, she promised to be with her good friends so that neither Jane nor Carol would have to go through this process alone.

Jane had always been an honest, direct person, but she had always been discreet about the specifics of her end-of-life philosophy. Once her plan was set, however, she became more open about her impending death, even with people with whom she had been less intimate in the past. Though many tried to talk her out of it at first, most of her good friends became convinced that she was doing what she needed to do. Since no one knew her exact plan, calls to her home often included a sigh of relief. "I wasn't sure if you would still be here."

Eventually a date was set. The timing was practical. Winter was approaching, so it was time to leave her country home in western New York. She did not want to travel to Arizona, and she was adamant about not moving in with friends in spite of genuine invitations.

On the day she had chosen, the three friends spent the day together. Although tension was in the air, much of the activity and conversation was mundane. Bills were paid, important documents were identified, and personal items were distributed. They had dinner together. Jane took a shower, and they watched television. Carol and Sarah waited in quiet anticipation for Jane to show them the way. Perhaps she would even change her mind.

Late that evening Jane told them she was ready. The medicine was prepared in applesauce, but it still tasted bitter. With great resolve, Jane swallowed all the pills without vomiting. She was unwavering and seemed peaceful. She rapidly became sleepy and tearfully said good-bye to Carol and Sarah, thanking them for being such good friends. She promised to let them know what life was like on the other side. She looked forward to returning to the twilight she had experienced once before, only this time not to return.

Jane entered a very deep sleep. Her respirations were shallow and her pulse was thready. She became completely unarousable. Unfortunately, five hours later she was still in limbo between life and death. Carol and Sarah did not know how to respond. Foremost in their mind was their commitment to Jane, who might be brain-damaged if she survived, and devastated if she regained consciousness. Jane had explained to them about the use of a plastic bag, which was suggested by the Hemlock Society for these circumstances. Although this prospect seemed gruesome and would be hard to live with, Carol and Sarah felt they had no choice. They knew that this intervention would not cause Jane further suffering, but they also realized that it would make their burden much heavier. It was a no-win situation. They had come this far; not abandoning their good friend was now their foremost responsibility.

They fulfilled their commitment by using the plastic bag. Jane died without struggling. They called Jane's local doctor and reported that she had died in her sleep after having been much sicker over the past several days. The doctor seemed mildly surprised, but he had also witnessed her hovering on the edge of requiring mechanical ventilation during her last hospitalization. He would call the undertaker and sign the death certificate. Jane was cremated so that there would be no trace of the process and no legal vulnerability for her close friends and her physician.

Thank God, Jane did not have to die alone. She was very fortunate to have friends who had the courage to listen and respond to her and did not turn back when they faced a terrible challenge at the very end. Her death was consistent with who she was as a person. She was not forced to endure more suffering and disability than she could tolerate. She was set free to go to a better place, and she went in peace.

Carol and Sarah were left trying to make sense of their participation in Jane's death. Because this act had to be carried out in secret, and there could be criminal repercussions, their grieving was made much more complex. Furthermore, the plastic bag had to leave an adverse imprint. There must be a better way.

Carol has thought extensively and felt deeply about her actions. Her retelling of Jane's story was filled with tears of joy and sadness. Carol waits patiently for Jane to give her a signal about what life is like on the "other side." She has no doubt that she fulfilled her commitment to her friend, whom she loved so dearly. Yet Carol is also angry that this process was made unnecessarily harsh and isolating by current legal restraints.

Sarah still doesn't talk much about it. Her faith in the hereafter is less strong, and because of her needs as a solver of problems she has lingering doubts about whether she did enough to try to dissuade Jane. Since she cannot talk openly about what actually happened, Sarah's ability to heal and grow from this experience has been thwarted. Sarah came through for her friends, but she may have been injured in the process.

Jane was very lucky to have such good friends. I hope they each make peace with their role in Jane's death. Without them her transition from this life to the next would have been much harsher and might have jeopardized the integrity so essential to her person. She would not have found an acceptable escape without their loving assistance and courage.

Commentary

1. *We are profoundly influenced by the deaths we have witnessed.* How those we love die becomes part of our core experience as human beings and influences how we see our own future. Jane's values and approach toward the end of her life were shaped in part by her work as a nurse. She listened to and learned from her terminally ill patients, taking their laments and their wish for death seriously. Because of this experience, she was able to speak openly to her friend Bill and listen when he talked about wanting to die. Though Jane had seen many "good deaths" in her work as a nurse, the more humiliating deaths haunted her. Jane had tried her best to respond to Bill's devastating disease near the end of his life, only to have him shoot himself in the head to "protect" her from legal vulnerability. This trauma made Jane, as well as Bill's wife and everyone who knew the circumstances of his death, more frightened about death than ever.

Carol and Sarah were willing to help Jane in part because they had the courage to listen when she talked about her current suffering and about the kind of future she wanted to avoid. They successfully helped Jane achieve a wished-for death without the humiliation and loss of control she feared, but the plastic bag they had to use at the very end undermined what would otherwise have been a very moving, positive experience. This stark image should have no place in a society that responds humanely to its dying; it reflects abandonment by the medical and legal professions and a desperate heroism by friends who refuse to turn their backs. As Carol and Sarah face death in their futures, images of Bill and Jane will reemerge that contain friendship, courage, and fear. One bad death powerfully influences all those who bear witness.

We must be much more creative in pursuing a broader range of paths by which people can complete their life story in ways consistent with their values and who they are as persons. There were no simple solutions for Bill or Jane. Yet forcing them to endure in a severely diminished state against their will seems cruel and unnecessary. Disintegration and humiliation threaten not only one's own life story but also the hopes and fears of close friends and family members. All those who witness bad deaths in which physicians were afraid to act must wonder about systems of medical ethics and law that glibly trade off the suffering of real people for the abstract good of society. How explicitly and forthrightly we handle these "rare" cases in which suffering is extreme at the very end in spite of excellent palliative care says a lot about us as a society and about medicine as a profession. Turning our backs on those few whose needs do not fit neatly into our current ethical framework undermines the excellent care we provide to the majority who are lucky enough to complete their life stories with their personhood intact.

2. *A patient's request for barbiturates in the final phase of illness must be addressed forthrightly.* Jane gave me every opportunity to carry out a covert conversation. In the United States we currently have a paradoxical situation according to which it is legally dangerous for physicians to give patients access to barbiturates if there is an explicit conversation about their potential use in overdose. The safest course is either to withhold the medicine no matter how terrible the patient's circumstances or to have an indirect, ambiguous conversation. "I need barbiturates to sleep." "Okay, but don't take too much or it could kill you." Such conversations are dangerous to patients as well as to the profes-

sion, for they undermine the trust and honesty essential to all medical decision making, particularly at the end of life. The doctor needs to know with certainty if the patient is requesting the barbiturates because of trouble sleeping or because the patient wants to have them available either in case future suffering becomes overwhelming or because the suffering is intolerable now and the patient wishes to die. Without explicit discussion, the opportunity to find other avenues to relieve suffering may be lost.

When a patient makes a request for help in dying, this should be seen as a cry for help, the meaning of which can be understood only through careful exploration. Giving a prescription for barbiturates without fully understanding why the request is coming at a particular point in time is just as bad as turning one's back. A humane and ethical system would take the legal threat out of the conversation and reinforce honesty and directness. There would be no tolerance for purposely ambiguous conversations, and even less for abandoning patients to act on their own. Giving barbiturate prescriptions to dying patients should be very rare, subject to the scrupulous safeguards of an open system, but not so impossible or risky that patients have to take matters violently into their own hands (Bill) or take an overdose without adequate medical backup (Jane), forcing family and friends to respond without medical guidance if things do not go as planned (Carol and Sarah).

3. *Laws prohibiting physician-assisted suicide are currently being challenged in state referendums and in federal courts.* Oregon recently became the first state in the United States to legalize physician-assisted suicide by narrowly passing a referendum entitled Proposition 16. Oregon's law allows physicians to openly prescribe barbiturates for their terminally ill patients who request them, subject to the following safeguards: (1) the patient must have a prognosis of six months or less; (2) the patient's request must be made in writing and must be repeated after a fifteen-day waiting period; (3) the patient must be rational and competent, his or her judgment not being distorted by clinical depression or other disorders; (4) a second medical opinion must be obtained; and (5) the patient must be capable of independently ingesting the medication. Notifica-

tion of the family is recommended but not required. The legalization of physician-assisted suicide that resulted from the referendum's passage is currently under challenge in the courts.

In Oregon the law has served as a wake-up call to the medical profession. Many hospitals across the state are suddenly finding funding for palliative care specialists and teams, and requests for teaching about pain management and hospice care within medical circles have never been higher. The referendum appears to have elicited an acknowledgment that the profession has not taken the needs of dying patients seriously enough. If this, along with giving more choice and control back to dying patients and their families, is the net result, then we should rapidly pass such a law in every state. If the constitutionality of the Oregon referendum is eventually upheld, then we will need to carefully research and monitor whether the obvious benefits of a more open process to patients like Jane, Bill, and Diane would outweigh the risks of subtle or explicit coercion.

The United States Court of Appeals in both the Ninth and the Second Circuit recently determined that state laws prohibiting physician-assisted suicide violate the U.S. Constitution. Almost overnight these decisions created the potential for a more open practice of physician-assisted suicide in the twelve states under their jurisdiction— California, Oregon, Washington, Idaho, Arizona, Montana, Nevada, Alaska, and Hawaii in the Ninth Circuit and New York, Vermont, and Connecticut in the Second Circuit. In *Compassion in Dying v. State of Washington*, the Ninth Circuit determined in an 8–3 decision that competent, terminally ill, suffering patients have a "constitutionally protected liberty interest in hastening what might otherwise be a protracted, undignified, and extremely painful death." The Second Circuit, in *Quill v. Vacco*, used different logic to reach a similar conclusion. Using an equal-protection argument, the court determined in a unanimous decision that it is unfair to allow some terminally ill suffering patients to die by choosing to stop life supports, whereas others whose suffering may be equal or even more severe but who have no life supports to discontinue are deprived of a similar option. In a supplementary opinion, Judge Calabresi suggested that the current laws prohibiting assisted suicide were not constructed to apply to modern medical decisions, in which the potential for a slow, agonizing death has increased significantly with advances in medical technology. He argued that rather than creating a new constitutionally protected liberty interest, state legislatures should be challenged to pass laws that take into account current clinical and legal realities regulating how doctors respond to terminally ill patients who are suffering severely and request assisted death.

Both circuit court decisions are being appealed to the United States Supreme Court. If the Supreme Court chooses to consider one or both of these cases, then the practice of physician-assisted death will remain underground until its legal status is firmly established. If the Court chooses not to consider these cases at the present time, then these practices will become legal in the twelve states under the jurisdiction of the two circuit courts. Each state will then have to determine how to regulate the practice. As suggested in both circuit court decisions, regulation should attempt to protect vulnerable populations but cannot be so restrictive that it makes access to a physician-assisted death prohibitive to those in need. Physician-assisted suicide has never been openly conducted in this country, so there is little infrastructure in place to oversee and study such practices. Since we have no experience under an open system, the importance of building in mechanisms for understanding and improving the practice over time cannot be overstated.

Speculation about the extent of the secret practice of physician-assisted death was recently clarified by a study of practicing physicians in Washington State.[3] They found that 12 percent of doctors received at least one genuine request for assisted suicide in the year studied, and an additional 4 percent received a request for euthanasia. Twenty-four percent of the doctors in each group provided the potentially lethal

3. A. L. Back et al., Physician-assisted suicide and euthanasia in Washington State: Patient requests and physician responses, *Journal of the American Medical Association* 275 (1996): 919–25.

medication in response to the patient's request. Consultations were infrequent, and none of the cases was reported as other than a natural death on the death certificate. Uncontrolled pain was rarely the sole reason for a request; more often the reason was a combination of physical, psychological, social, and existential suffering. This study confirms that the secret practice of physician-assisted death is not rare, that undertreated pain is not the predominant driving force, and that current practices are completely unregulated. It seems clear that a more open system would be safer and more predictable for patients than the current system of looking the other way.

If we are to extend ourselves as a compassionate society to openly sanction physician-assisted suicide as the intervention of last resort, we must not allow our ambivalence about the act to let us ignore the circumstances when it does not work. If passing such laws is an ultimate expression of solidarity with patients who have suffered too much, we must specifically consider cases like Jane's, in which the drugs are ineffective or unanticipated complications develop. Physicians who are willing to provide such assistance must be required to be available to support the patient and family and to be responsive if problems arise. No one should be forced to die alone, or to die with a plastic bag over his or her head, because we are afraid to fully address the practical implications of what we are allowing.

References

Influence of Witnessing

American Board of Internal Medicine. *Caring for the Dying—Identification and Promotion of Physician Competency: Personal Narratives.* Philadelphia, 1996.

Eddy, D. M. A conversation with my mother. *Journal of the American Medical Association* 272 (1994): 179–81.

Edwards, M. J., and S. W. Tolle. Disconnecting a ventilator at the request of a patient who knows he will then die: The doctor's anguish. *Annals of Internal Medicine* 117 (1992): 254–56.

Loxterkamp, D. A good death is hard to find: Preliminary reports of a hospice doctor. *Journal of the American Board of Family Practice* 6 (1993): 415–17.

Nuland, S. B. *How We Die: Reflections on Life's Final Chapter.* New York: Knopf, 1994.

Quill, T. E. Death and dignity: A case of individualized decision making. *New England Journal of Medicine* 324 (1991): 691–94.

Rollin, B. *Last Wish.* New York: Warner Books, 1985.

Shavelson, L. *A Chosen Death: The Dying Confront Assisted Suicide.* New York: Simon & Schuster, 1995.

Responding to Requests for Physician-Assisted Death

Baile, W. F., J. R. DiMaggio, D. V. Schapira, and J. S. Janofsky. The request for assistance in dying: The need for psychiatric consultation. *Cancer* 72 (1993): 2786–91.

Block, S. D., and J. A. Billings. Patient requests to hasten death: Evaluation and management in terminal care. *Archives of Internal Medicine* 154 (1994): 2039–47.

Gert, B., J. L. Bernat, and R. P. Mogielnicki. Distinguishing between patient's refusals and requests. *Hastings Center Report*, July–August 1994, 13–15.

Quill, T. E. Doctor, I want to die. Will you help me? *Journal of the American Medical Association* 270 (1993): 870–73.

Quill, T. E., and R. V. Brody. "You promised me I wouldn't die like this": A bad death as a medical emergency. *Archives of Internal Medicine* 155 (1995): 1250–54.

Rie, M. A. The limits of a wish. *Hastings Center Report*, July–August 1991, 24–27.

Legal Challenges

Alpers, A., and B. Lo. Physician-assisted suicide in Oregon: A bold experiment. *Journal of the American Medical Association* 274 (1995): 483–87.

Annas, G. J. Death by prescription: The Oregon initiative. *New England Journal of Medicine* 331 (1994): 1240–43.

Back, A. L., J. I. Wallace, H. E. Starks, and R. A. Pearlman. Physician-assisted suicide and euthanasia in Washington State: Patient requests and physician responses. *Journal of the American Medical Association* 275 (1996): 919–25.

Baron, C. H., C. Bergstresser, D. W. Brock, G. F. Cole, N. S. Dorfman, J. A. Johnson, L. E. Schnipper, J. Vorenberg, and S. W. Wanzer. Statute: A Model state act to authorize and regulate physician-assisted suicide. *Harvard Journal on Legislation* 32 (1996): 1–34.

Compassion in Dying v. State of Washington No. 94–35534, 1996 WL 94848 (9th Cir., 6 March 1996).

Lee, M. A., and S. W. Tolle. Oregon's assisted suicide vote: The silver lining. *Annals of Internal Medicine* 124 (1996): 267–69.

Quill v. Vacco (State of New York), No. 95–7028 (2d Cir., 9 April 1996).

Chapter 9

Loving Assistance

JULES HAD A planned death, down to the last detail. He chose late April, after taxes were due. In addition to carefully saying all his goodbyes, he wanted to make sure the year's finances were in order. He would have loved to live longer, but his future held only further deterioration. He had already held on much longer than he ever thought he could. Jules died in his own home surrounded by devoted family and friends, his doctor by his side providing assistance and technical advice. Even the doctor had a colleague present for her support. No one was alone. Everyone felt loved and cared for. It was a sad but joyous occasion. Jules would be missed as a father, husband, and friend, but he was also being set free from his deteriorating body, which was now a fragile shell of its former self.

Could this be a true story? Given the current legal fears and uncertainties under which dying patients, their families, and physicians are often forced to operate, how could this open, caring environment be created? Perhaps it is a fictional rendition of how dying could be in this country, with decisions made out in the open by people who care deeply about one another and are not afraid to face up to the cruelty disease sometimes inflicts. Jules's story is in fact true. His death reflects a moment in time when the lives of a diverse array of individuals briefly intersected to help Jules through the biggest challenge of his life. To explain Jules's final chapter, I should start closer to the beginning.

Jules had deep blue eyes and a warm, engaging smile that put one immediately at ease. He was articulate and engaging, a good listener who was not afraid to speak his mind. His frame was large and muscular. Physical prowess was part of his self-definition, both at home and on the job. He spent time and energy exercising his intelligence and spirit as well as his body. His depth of thought and warm personality allowed people to quickly connect with him. He had a particular love for good food and wine. His vivid descriptions of a wonderful meal could stimulate the senses and the imagination. He worked in human resources, a perfect medium for his talents. Both management and staff felt that he could represent them and look out for their interests.

Although Jules was very attractive to women, he did not settle down until he met Judith, when they were both in their mid-thirties. Judith was also strong willed and caring. She thought she might never fall fully in love or get married, but in Jules she finally found a soul mate. Judith had spent most of her professional life working in a neurology clinic for patients with amyotrophic lateral sclerosis (ALS, or Lou Gerhig's disease). She loved her work and was dedicated to the patients, whom she would follow through their slow but inevitable decline. More than most, she was daily reminded at work that life can be short and dying can sometimes occur in small, relentless increments rather than discrete events. Judith and Jules shared many interests, including fine food and travel. They both had a serious, introspective side. Jules's inward journey took him to the Gestalt Institute and Tavastock, among other places. Even before Jules became sick, he and Judith had long talks about life and death, as well as their concern about excessive suffering near the end of life. They promised to help each other find death if the need arose. It was part of their commitment to each other.

Jules and Judith dated and then lived together for several years before getting married. One year after their marriage their son Stefan was born. Jules loved all aspects of fatherhood, from cuddling to storytelling to changing diapers. Stefan and Jules did everything together; they were always on the go, enjoying every minute. Although with both parents working and life jam-packed, Jules found that the exhilaration and intimacy far outweighed the demands. Because Judith was by then over forty, they knew that if they wanted more children they had to act swiftly or her biological clock would run out. When she again became pregnant, they decided on amniocentesis because the risk of genetic defects was relatively high. Sadly, the amniocentesis showed genetic markers of Down's syndrome. After agonizing and soul-searching, they decided that Judith would have an abortion. They felt strongly that they were doing the right thing for themselves and for their potentially unborn baby, but they also lost a piece of themselves in the process. They would try again, but their grief was deep and lasting.

Tragically, the same genetic problem showed up with the next pregnancy. Their decision was the same, and the darkness grew. The dream of a larger family was again thwarted. If only they had met earlier in life, things would have been different. Although they still found great joy in each other and in their son, there was an empty place in their life, a shadow of what might have been.

The first sign of Jules's illness came in 1990, on the heels of these losses. They had been married three years and Stefan was two years old. The first symptoms seemed relatively innocent. Jules always had a project. At the time he was vigorously sanding, putting the finishing touches on the summer cottage he had helped to build. His hands cramped so severely that he was unable to drive home. He called Judith to tell her he would be late. His strength gradually returned, and by morning his hands were back to normal. It was just one of life's little mysteries that scare us but do not mean a great deal. Or so they thought.

Over the next six months Jules continued to have minor problems with strength and coordination in his hands. His deficit was most evident whenever he did physically demanding projects. His internist eventually arranged a neurological consultation. A relatively mild, asymmetric weakness was found in Jules's hands. The rest of his physical exam seemed normal. Formal nerve conduction testing was inconclusive.

"Have you ever had polio?"

"No."

"Did you have any exposure to toxins in your work?"

"No."

"Has anyone in the family in prior generations had anything similar?"

"No."

The list of blind alleys seemed endless.

"What could it be?" they finally asked, not sure they wanted to hear the answer.

"I am not sure. It could be some form of ALS, post-polio syndrome, or some ill-defined neuropathy. Only time will tell."

Oh, my God! Their minds were reeling, but they remained silent. This must be some kind of cosmic joke! Judith had spent much of her adult life caring for patients with ALS, nurturing them through one of the cruelest of illnesses. How different things appeared from the other side of the looking glass! Life couldn't be that perverse! Perhaps it was only a neuropathy! This couldn't be happening to them!

ALS comes in many forms and progresses at different rates. There is no cure, and no way to slow the progression. Treatment consists largely in anticipating and responding to complications as they inevitably occur. ALS is characterized by its ability to damage both peripheral and central nerves, although brain cognition remains fully normal. The peripheral muscles lose their bulk and strength from lack of nerve stimulation, so one gradually loses the ability to walk and to manipulate one's environment with one's arms and hands. The ability to breathe, speak, and even eat independently is eventually compromised such that one cannot survive without breathing machines, feeding tubes, and constant medical supervision. All the while the mind remains completely intact and fully functional. It is hard to imagine this kind of deterioration unless you have personally witnessed it. Sometimes the lack of full knowledge can be kind. Most individuals make gradual adjustments over time that would have been unthinkable if they had to be made all at once. The time course is variable, sometimes progressing over months, at other times over many years.

Having spent the better part of twenty years working in an ALS clinic, Judith did not have the luxury of being naive or uninformed. Although somewhere in her subconscious ALS remained a possibility, she was able to keep it at bay most of the time. Jules was too healthy for this kind of disease, too vibrant, too full of life. Their life together was just getting started; there was so much they had yet to experience. Besides, his illness had too many atypical features and he was too young. Perhaps if they didn't think too much about it, it would go away. At times like this some degree of denial can be a good friend.

Judith's denial lasted six months. Jules gradually had to give up doing projects that required considerable upper-body strength. His legs became numb whenever he walked long distances. He began to lose his robust physique and found himself exhausted by the workday. He eventually had trouble buttoning his clothes and doing other tasks that required fine motor dexterity. To someone who had not seen him in a few months the physical changes were obvious, but they can still sneak up on you if you live with them day to day.

Reality came crashing down on Judith during a subsequent visit to the neurologist. Jules had now clearly developed hyperreflexia (a sign of upper motor neuron problems) along with weakness and quivering of the muscles (signs of lower motor neuron dysfunction). This combination of findings was a clear sign to her of ALS. *Oh, my God! Jules really has ALS!* The anguish permeated all aspects of Judith's being. *He really has it! What are we going to do?* It was as if she were understanding Jules's condition for the first time and putting it in the context of all the other patients she had known over the years.

As if to confound the drastic turn that their life was taking, Judith became pregnant again one month later. Reeling from their awareness about Jules's diagnosis, they did not have the emotional energy to deal with another wrenching decision. Judith would get an abortion. How could they have a baby, given the uncertainty of Jules's future? Besides, the odds of the genetic defect repeating itself were very high given Judith's age and their two recent pregnancies. Judith went to her obstetrician, who convinced them to think things over and consider having amniocentesis before making a final decision. They cautiously waited and eventually even dared to be a little hopeful. Their son Stefan predicted the baby would be a healthy girl. To their joy and surprise, the amniocentesis proved him right on both counts. Four and one-half months later Sarah was born, as normal as she could be.

During Stefan's delivery Jules had been an active partner in every way. In the months before Sarah's birth Jules's condition had progressed dramatically. His gait was now unsteady and he had difficulty even taking care of his own personal needs, much less those of the rest of the family. In the birthing room this time Jules lay at Judith's side on his own gurney, providing emotional support but too weak to hold the baby. Storm clouds were all around, but it was still a joyous occasion. Sarah was their "miracle baby," a gift they had not dared to hope for in the midst of their tragedy.

Jules's ALS did not subsequently follow an indolent course. He continued to work full-time, but all he could do when he got home was gather strength for the next day. He lost more than fifty pounds, and walking short distances exhausted him. His eloquent speech was reduced to a soft, halting staccato. He learned how to communicate cryptically, lest he become exhausted simply by the effort of talking. Making it to the bathroom became increasingly difficult; he had to leave with time to spare or risk losing control of his urine en route. He had long since given up on buttons, securing all of his clothing with Velcro straps. Judith had also obtained every conceivable assistive device. Several months after Sarah was born, Jules finally decided to retire. Work was taking too much out of him. Although work had always been an informing theme in his life, retiring would allow him to save what little energy he had for Judith and the children. He had continued working much longer than he should have from a medical point of view. Stopping was a painful admission of just how debilitated he had become.

Jules and Judith began to talk openly about his dying and about how much deterioration he would be willing to tolerate. His energy had improved since his retirement, and he still found great joy in caring for the children and sharing his life with Judith. But there would be limits. Jules felt that he would hang on as long as he could but stop short of breathing machines and feeding tubes. When he could no longer breathe and eat on his own, he would call it quits. He and Judith began to collect information about methods for achieving a humane death, both from Judith's colleagues, who were receptive to the inquiry, and from the Hemlock Society. As part of this preparation, Jules made a videotape for each of his children to tell them how much he loved them, how much he wished he could watch them grow up, and that he would always be with them in spirit if not in body. Jules knew he would deteriorate to the point where his speech would be unintelligible. He wanted to leave his children with a remembrance of him speaking personally about his love.

Jules's doctors had a hard time acknowledging his deterioration. His internist would meet with him and ignore or minimize what was happening. "Everything looked good." Since Jules was in the habit of confronting even the hardest of problems head on, he found this superficial encouragement infuriating. His neurologist was a personal friend of Judith's. He initially allowed Jules considerable flexibility in controlling his own care, even meeting him socially for a drink rather than having appointments at the neurologic clinic. Although the neurologist seemed to share Jules's discouragement about his deterioration, he felt the need to constantly encourage him to keep fighting. Later, when Jules would talk about wanting to die, the neurologist vehemently tried to talk him out of it. Others with ALS had learned how to cope with so much less. Depression must be clouding his judgment. Surely, with all his inner strengths, intelligence, and family support, Jules too could learn to adapt. Their work together eventually stopped feeling like a collaboration and took on the character of a struggle for control over Jules's future.

In early 1993 Jules became so weak that his breathing was too shallow to sustain him and he was admitted to the hospital for evaluation. Formal pulmonary function testing showed that his breathing capacity was dangerously limited and he was not getting enough oxygen. A tracheostomy (a hole in the throat through which one can breath and be attached to a breathing machine) was recommended. Delay would be dangerous and possibly lethal. The doctors wanted his consent, not a lengthy discussion about whether Jules wanted to cross this threshold. Jules felt pushed to make a decision. The more they pressured him, the more he dug in his heels. He eventually decided to go home before making up his mind.

Jules left the hospital knowing he had no good choices. Without treatment he would gradually suffocate. No alternative to the tracheostomy and the breathing machine had been presented. The possibility of having his shortness of breath comforted with morphine and being "allowed to die" had not been explored. Yet, in truth, even if morphine sedation had been offered, Jules was not yet ready to die. He still had wonderful, intimate times with Stefan and Sarah, and he could savor small amounts of fine food in shared meals with Judith. Life had become very restricted, but it was still worth living in spite of all of its limitations. He simply wanted to have a serious voice in what was happening to him.

Jules chose to go back to the hospital and have the tracheostomy. Unfortunately, he developed pneumonia postoperatively. He was in the hospital for over a month, an experience he found excruciating. Because his speech was very slow, many on the staff spoke to him in a patronizing way. People made assumptions and decisions that seemed to discount him as a person. Jules had never been treated this way before, and he found the lack of respect and understanding both demoralizing and frightening. He stopped fighting and lay passively in bed for days at a time. His dwindling strength would never recover from the days of inactivity. He eventually left the hospital, vowing never to return. He would sooner die than go back. He also began to search for a physician who would value partnership more than control, one who would respect him in spite of his declining physical abilities. It was then that Jules met Betty.

Betty is a primary care physician who came to the United States by way of Beer Sheva, Israel, where she received her initial training. Her mentors in Israel were very knowledgeable, caring physicians with a paternalistic orientation who engaged deeply with their patients. Medicine in Israel is guided almost exclusively by an all-out fight for life. The notion of patients taking charge toward the end, setting limits on this heroic battle, is an anathema. Patients' wishes for less than the most aggressive care are frequently overridden, albeit with beneficent intent. Betty arrived in Rochester highly proficient in the fight for life, but in her subsequent training she learned about an approach to medical care that genuinely encouraged patients to become actively involved. She also learned about comfort-oriented care as a humane alternative for dying patients, emphasizing quality of life more than quantity. Betty mastered both the technical and the interpersonal skills needed to make comfort-oriented care a reality for most of her dying patients. After she completed her fellowship, she joined me in practice and developed a devoted cadre of patients. But she had never before had a relationship with a patient like Jules, who had an extremely strong sense of self, clearly articulated wishes, and a vexing, ultimately fatal disease. Working with Jules, Betty continued her own personal journey, learning about the implications of working in partnership with people who face devastating illness.

From the outset, Jules, Judith, and Betty had a special relationship. Betty would allow Jules to talk openly about his hopes and fears. Fearing suffocation, Jules had struggled to breathe for a long period of time before his tracheostomy. He was now more afraid of further physical disintegration than he was of death. He was, however, willing to withstand his current profound losses and continue the fight primarily because of his children. He had changed his mind about having a tracheostomy and going on a ventilator, but he would draw the line at having artificial feeding. Jules loved food, and he would remain a gourmet until the bitter end. "No feeding tube. When I get to that point, I will call it quits." Betty had never encountered anyone who was so articulate and open about death. She had her own anxiety about death, and she was uncertain how far a physician should go to relieve a patient's suffering. Yet Betty was still willing to articulate her commitment to Jules: "When the time comes for you to die, and you are completely sure, I will be there for you and help you as best I can." For both Jules and Judith, this commitment was both reassuring and liberating, a striking contrast with the encounters they had had with previous physicians, who would either avoid the issue entirely or discourage such thinking.

Jules and Betty had their initial meeting in her office; however, the trip had been so exhausting for Jules that subsequent visits took place in his home. Betty became a friend as well as physician, visiting regularly so that they could get to know one another. Unfortunately, their first medical crisis was not far away.

Jules still loved the taste and smell of good food. Even though he had great difficulty chewing and swallowing, he and Judith still managed to share elegant meals complete with tastes of special wine. Food would sometimes get stuck in Jules's throat, and he would gasp for air as his weakened cough would try to clear it. Meals frequently left him exhausted. Yet, the taste, smell, and preparation of fine food were part of his core being. Maintaining these pleasures remained essential despite the increasing risk of developing pneumonia from aspiration.

I wish I could report that it was a wonderful meal or a sip of special wine that accidentally got into Jules's lungs. Instead, it was a McDonald's hamburger eaten with his children. When Betty saw him, he had a high fever and was struggling to breathe. Although he did not want to go to the hospital, he also was not ready to die. After an intense negotiation, he agreed to go to the emergency department for a chest x-ray, a test of the oxygen in his blood, and cultures of his blood and sputum.

Jules almost died twice in the next several days. In the emergency department his blood pressure dropped while his blood was being drawn. Having no acceptable alternatives, he allowed himself to be admitted to the intensive care unit for the treatment of pneumonia. He felt terribly anxious and out of control, so he was given a mild sedative, which dangerously suppressed his frail respiratory drive. For a short while his body did not get enough oxygen. No one noticed, and he was too impaired to call out. His condition was very fragile, and he was so dependent on others that even a minor misstep could be a matter of life and death.

Because of the hectic pace of the intensive care unit, his limited ability to communicate left him largely at the mercy of the doctors and nurses. He felt trapped, vulnerable, and at times hopeless about his future. When Judith visited, sometimes all Jules could do was sob uncontrollably. He felt humiliated and defeated. He even consented to the temporary use of a feeding tube because he felt that otherwise he would never get home. It could be discontinued at any time. Jules was eventually discharged with a complicated plan of home supports. He again vowed never to return to the hospital. He knew he would die soon, and he didn't want to die with his body and soul in the hands of people who didn't know him.

Jules had always been a deep thinker and a skilled communicator. He enjoyed exploring ideas, and he was known for his incisive intellect, honesty, and genuineness. As his illness progressed, his once articulate speech became painfully slow, sometimes unintelligible. He was eventually reduced to using a letter board. As his hands became weaker, he and Judith learned how to use the device together like a Ouija board. She would follow his subtle cues about where to stop. Sophisticated exchanges that in the past would have taken a matter of minutes now took hours of painstaking cooperation and partnership. Jules's mind was still fully active and alert, but it was trapped in a body that could barely speak, much less move. Endless time and patience were needed for Judith to understand what Jules needed. She would then advocate for him in the fast-paced world that had little ability to listen in slow motion.

Jules was also a very private person. With his ALS, his privacy was invaded on all fronts. He eventually needed assistance with all bodily functions, from bathing to toileting to moving from his bed to the chair. Some home health aides and nurses had a gift for making this process as comfortable and dignified as possible, but others treated him roughly or, even worse, in a demeaning way. Judith made every effort to surround him with caring, respectful persons, but he needed care twenty-four hours a day, seven days a week. The stream of strangers was relentless. Some would become intimate friends, and others bitter enemies. In addition, his private thoughts now also had to become more public. Since he literally could not act in any way on his own, he had to share his most intimate thoughts with Judith, and then together they would decide how to proceed. Since each conversation might take several hours, they often had to ask the nurses or aides to leave so that they could talk. His life was no longer his own, and his integrity as a person was hanging by a thread. Judith was his lifeline and protector.

The losses and frustrations were at times overwhelming, but there remained some wonderful moments. Jules liked nothing better than to lie in his bed watching television with Stefan and Sarah. They were like three peas in a pod during those times, feeling close and connected, completely at peace with the world. Jules kept to a routine. He spent a large part of each day in a chair that placed him in the center of all household activities. The children could play all around him, and he could see and participate in everything. Although he regretted that he couldn't change Sarah's diapers or clip her little nails, as he had done for Stefan, he loved watching them interact with the world. Fathering became his greatest joy, and the children felt his closeness in spite of his limitations. A birdfeeder was placed in a window near his chair, and they loved to watch the wide variety of birds come and visit.

Jules remained very communicative at times in spite of his deficits. He learned to be very direct and cryptic, communicating with his eyes, blowing a kiss, or saying "I love you." One stopped mincing words in such a situation. He and Judith developed a gallows humor, joking about unhooking his respirator as a way of resolving their disputes. Although he had then lost over one hundred pounds and was a shadow of his former self, Jules still had a powerful presence. He could communicate feelings with his bright blue eyes and gestures. To express his more complicated thoughts, Judith had become his voice. Because of these joys, he hung on to life much longer than he had thought he would.

Swallowing continued to be a major problem for Jules after he left the hospital. He could not eat enough to sustain himself. The ordeal of trying to chew and swallow exhausted him, and there was a constant risk of getting food into his lungs. The artificial feeding he was getting through his nasogastric tube helped to stem his weight loss and malnutrition. Betty eventually convinced Jules to have a tube placed directly into his stomach. If he wanted to eat food regularly through his mouth, he still could, but he would not have to struggle to maintain all his nutritional needs. Although he had vowed to stop treatment at this point, he decided to give it a try. Even though much of his life seemed tortured and meaningless, he was not ready to leave the joys that he still found in his young family. Since Jules remained adamant about avoiding hospitalization, Betty arranged to have the tube put in as an outpatient procedure.

The tube was inserted without a hitch, and Jules returned home the same day. It functioned perfectly, and his nutritional status continued to improve. Unfortunately, Jules subsequently became very discouraged. The fight to keep eating and the enjoyment of food had been symbolically important, and giving in to the tube had left him spiritually and emotionally depleted. Jules was used to structure, yet he gave up on his routine of getting up every morning. He would stay in bed until late in the day, and he became detached from the joys of his family and the household financial decisions, which had helped to sustain him. This marked a very dark period in Jules's illness. Judith and Betty could not find the key to pull him out of it. His malnutrition was improving, but as a person he was getting much worse. His suffering at this point was as much existential as physical. In spite of being surrounded by caring family and receiving the best of palliative care, he had reached the point of no return. He angrily refused antidepressant medication when it was recommended by his neurologist. This was not a mental problem. He was trapped in a body that had betrayed him, and he had no prospect of getting better. He had adjusted and adapted all that he could. He then recalled what Betty had promised him: "When it all gets to be too much, I will be there for you. I will do whatever you need me to." He could feel his spirit reviving.

In December Jules began to communicate with Judith about how he had reached the end of his rope. As he openly explored the possibility of dying, his energy and mood improved. He had initially thought he would never go onto a respirator or have a feeding tube, but he had given both a try. He did not regret these decisions. He had gained precious time, but these life-sustaining treatments no longer had value to him. Jules felt a profound sadness at having to leave Judith and the children. They had become his heart and soul during the overwhelming loss and degradation of the past year, but he now felt that the burdens outweighed the rewards for all of them. Judith told Jules that, in spite of the hardships, she would rather he live but that she would respect and support his decision. He initially chose February, but Judith asked him to wait until after Sarah's second birthday. Jules eventually settled on a date late in April, after tax day, so that all of their financial affairs would be in order. Once the date was set, he didn't waiver. "I have never felt this free," he would say.

Jules and Judith discussed the issue thoroughly before they shared his thinking with Betty. "I have never felt more anxious," Betty would report in retrospect. She initially challenged the decision from as many angles as possible. He wasn't having any physical pain, and his depression had lifted. There was an excellent supportive program at home, and Judith was more than willing to continue to provide care and coordination. Because of their generous major medical insurance policy, Jules could have had six more years of twenty-four-hour-a-day nursing coverage without touching their personal financial resources. After exploring the decision repeatedly with Jules and Judith, Betty finally accepted that he had thoroughly thought through the matter. Besides, they had plenty of time to reconsider over the next four months. She hoped he would change his mind.

Betty was unwavering in her commitment to Jules, but she was unsure at a practical level how to ensure his comfort after taking him off his respirator. She knew Jules was afraid of suffocation, and she had promised not to let that happen. She was not certain whether the law required that he struggle before she sedated him or whether she could give him a large dose of medicine before taking him off the respirator so that he would not suffer at all. The latter seemed more humane but frighteningly close to euthanasia. She would have to explore the legal implications and look for clinical precedents. Just as important, she would have to search her own soul to be sure that she could live with such an act. As profound as her commitment was to Jules, this was new territory for her and she found it frightening. Fortunately, she had time to prepare herself.

Betty quietly consulted with colleagues who had experience in palliative care, ethics, law, and neurology. She learned that taking patients off of life-sustaining treatment is both morally and legally acceptable. Competent patients have the right to stop unwanted treatment even if they will die as a result of that decision, and there was no doubt about Jules's competence. She got practical guidance concerning how much sedation to give him so that he wouldn't struggle when he was taken off the respirator. More than one well-intentioned physician had under-dermedicated such a patient, with the result that the patient was gasping for air before finally dying. In order to stay within the confines of the "double effect," the physician's intention must be to prevent the suffering that comes from suffocation and not to hasten death, but practically the physician must give a large dose of sedatives before removing the respirator in order to prevent the struggle. Betty asked about exact doses and backup plans so that she would be prepared for all eventualities.

Once she had researched and settled the legal and clinical questions to the best of her ability, Betty still had to work on her own inner issues. Although she was not an observant Jew, this act was diametrically opposed to the training she had received in Israel. Not entirely comfortable with death, she had often anguished when it was time to let go of dying patients. As she explored her own fears and the experiences of others, Betty struggled with fundamental questions. Were there limits to patient empowerment? What would she do in Jules's situation? Should this really be his choice to make? Should physicians ever override the decisions of dying patients? Was this level of intimacy with a suffering person healthy for her? Betty was unable to answer all of her questions. Her depth as a human being and her ability to administer to the dying, however, grew through the process.

Jules and Judith struggled over how to prepare their children. Should they tell them about the plan or keep it a secret? Leaving the children was the saddest part for Jules. He yearned to see them grow up and to remain an ongoing part of their lives. In anticipation of his death, he had videotaped messages for them when he was better able to talk. Jules and Judith elicited the help of a child psychologist who had expertise in bereavement. "Daddy will be leaving because he is very sick and he isn't going to get better. He is like a bird trapped in a cage. When he dies, it will be like setting the bird free. Daddy has been trapped in his sick body too long, and he needs to go. He loves you very much, and he will always love you." Who knows how these metaphors are understood in the minds and hearts of young children? They knew they were loved and that their Daddy was dying because he was sick, not because of them.

In the months preceding tax time Betty nurtured Jules through several life-threatening infections. He stayed at home, took antibiotics, and, surprisingly, survived. Jules remained generally optimistic and steadfast about his chosen course. Betty constantly reminded him that he could change his mind at any time, up to and including the last minute. In response, Jules would look up at her, smile, and say, "I love you too." "Are you afraid?" Betty would ask. "No," Jules would respond. "I have always been alone." Jules was a deep existential thinker through to the end. With the help of Judith and her mother, Jules was able to write letters to special people in his life, and a steady stream of friends came to say good-bye. Their closest family and friends were invited to be present. Betty would have one of her colleagues with her for moral and practical support. It would be a festive occasion—a bittersweet celebration. Jules asked that some special port he had been saving for Stefan's graduation from college be shared to commemorate the occasion.

Betty said in a later interview, "Something about knowing the time it was going to happen was eerie. The way life is arranged, none of us knows our moment of death. Our lives were traveling in a continuum marked by a specific time. There was something surreal about knowing the date and time. I kept thinking on Saturday morning about the hours going away. He was going to be dead in eight hours, in seven hours, in six hours . . . The people around me who knew all said a prayer at the time I said that Jules was going to die. I had gone to dinner with my closest friends, and when I left, they just sat there in complete silence, praying for him in some way. When I got there, the kitchen counter was filled with pictures of Jules—a collage of work pictures, wedding pictures, Jules as a young man and as a father. Empty wine glasses were out, along with a bottle of port that was to be opened when he died. They were reminiscing, laughing and telling stories. Jules was in the bedroom in his own bed, where he had not slept in months." He had selected some New Age music for the occasion, sounds from the Amazon rainforest, which everyone but Jules secretly disliked. Judith had spent much of the day frantically running from one task to another before she was finally able to settle down. When Betty arrived, Judith and her mother were stroking Jules's forehead as they talked quietly together.

"Are you sure you want to go through with this?" Betty asked.

"Yes," Jules nodded.

"We can open up the bottle of port anyway."

"No."

"You can still change your mind."

Jules looked up at Betty with his bright blue eyes and then moved his head back and forth like a fledgling bird.

It was time to set him free.

Betty mixed a substantial number of the barbiturate pills with a liquid and used a large syringe to administer the mixture through the feeding tube. Jules fell quickly into a deep sleep. One of Betty's practice partners arrived, and it turned out that he and Jules had been neighbors in the past. It was a small world that night; many lifelines were crossing at the same time and place. About twenty minutes later Judith took him off the respirator, fulfilling her promise to set him free when his time came. He was surrounded by loving family, dying in a way of his own choosing. Everyone present had made a peace with his decision. He lay there, quiet and motionless. His ordeal would soon be over. About ten minutes later the tranquility was broken when Jules grimaced and sighed! Everyone panicked! We had promised him he would not struggle! Although this might have been some involuntary agonal movement, he was temporarily put back on the breathing machine and more sedation was administered. Shortly thereafter he was again removed. This time there was no struggle. Everyone was supported, and no one was alone. There were tears of joy and sadness. He was moving on to a better place. As Judith's mother said, "There is nothing sad about him leaving that old, decaying body."

About thirty minutes later Betty declared that Jules was dead. The port was opened and everyone shared a toast. Somebody asked, "Now can we turn that damn music off?" and they all shared a laugh at Jules's expense. They had all witnessed the most profound of experiences and were richer for it.

The once mighty, now scrawny bird was finally flying free of his cage.

Commentary

1. *Medical decisions that end life, be they direct or indirect, intended or not, should always be challenging.* Someone's life hangs in the balance. Decisions to end life should be made with the utmost care, out in the open, involving the most experienced professionals. There is no turning back once these acts are carried out. The most challenging part should be ensuring that the patient is ready to die and that all palliative care alternatives have been adequately explored. The decision should be made jointly by the patient and the physician, usually involving the closest family and friends, depending on the patient's situation and preferences. External consultants should provide an unbiased perspective. Once the decision is made, the method used is relatively unimportant

from a moral point of view, provided it is effective, humane, and consistent with the values of the patient and the doctor.

In this particular case, Jules was oddly lucky that he had a life-sustaining treatment (his breathing machine) to stop. Because of this, a large dose of barbiturates or opioids could then be openly given by the doctor to prevent feelings of suffocation. Yet the specifics of the act and the ambiguity of the law left Betty confused. Did she have to wait for Jules to begin to flail before giving the barbiturate? If she gave it prophylactically, how big a dose should she give? If she gave a big enough dose to make sure that he did not struggle (as she should from a moral point of view), might she not be second-guessed legally for having euthanized Jules? Betty consulted other physicians about her responsibilities and about the practicalities of dosing, but she gave Jules only a moderate amount of barbiturates, which may have been the reason for his frightening gasp in the middle of what was otherwise an ideally peaceful process. She competently responded to this mini-crisis by giving him more sedation, but one lesson she learned was that "if I ever have to do this again, I will give enough sedation." Often, doctors undermedicate dying patients' pain or shortness of breath because of the legal risks (both exaggerated and real) associated with overmedicating. Since the doses of medicines required in the dying process are often well above usual range, it is no surprise that doctors too frequently err on the legally safe but morally suspect side of undermedicating.

2. *Jules's death illustrates the potential beauty of a more open, planned process.* No one wanted Jules to die, but all those close to him had ample opportunity to come to grips with his decision. To say he had not suffered enough would be preposterous. His decision to discontinue the ventilator gave him back control and hope, and his energy and engagement improved over his last four months. Although he was unwavering in his decision to let go, he took antibiotics several times to prolong his life during that period. Jules and Judith carefully prepared their children, with professional assistance. Leaving his children was extremely painful, but Jules hated the way his illness dominated all of

their lives. Although his family gave him clear, consistent messages that having him present was well worth all the struggle, Jules knew in his own heart that it was time to go. With the help of Judith and his mother-in-law, Jules was able to say good-bye to friends and family.

Unlike the chaotic processes that are all too familiar both in the hospital and at home, Jules's death was a meaningful ceremony. He was surrounded by those he loved, and many others who knew the time were there in spirit. Pictures reflecting his life dotted his landscape, and music of his choosing was playing in the background. He was being stroked and loved by those he cared about most, and his doctor was at his side to provide technical assistance and advice if anything went awry. When the minor crisis arose with Jules's agonal gasp, Betty was there to help respond. It did not undermine the confidence that they were witnessing a truly beautiful process. All who were present knew they were privileged to be there. It will stay with them forever. Jules's death illustrates the potential of a planned death, although it would not have happened in today's uncertain environment without the presence of exceptional people.

Jules's death was very life affirming. No one was alone. Everyone, including the doctor, had a shoulder to cry on. The process was profound, moving, and out in the open, not shrouded in secrecy or in legal uncertainty. It was hard enough without that added burden. Not only could people support one another while they were there but they could freely discuss their participation afterward without fear of legal recrimination. Those who were present will share a lifelong bond. Judith and her mother have subsequently become Betty's patients, they feel a connection that goes well beyond most doctor-patient relationships.

Having never assisted in such a death, Betty was anxious until the very end. She lost sleep and struggled with her role and responsibilities. When I asked if she continued to struggle afterward or had any doubts, she answered, "Not one, although I hope I don't have to go through this again."

3. *The real medical heroes in the care of the dying are the many doctors and*

nurses working in primary care, hospice, oncology, geriatrics, and nursing homes and with AIDS patients who seek to empower their patients throughout the last phase of their lives. End-of-life struggles sometimes involve a desperate fight for life in spite of very poor odds and other times include helping patients find a way to die that is consistent with their own values. Doing this work properly requires coming to know patients personally and allowing them as full an expression as possible in spite of the clinical circumstances. It is a commitment to face the unknowable future together in partnership. On rare occasions it may include assisting a patient to die when all other avenues have been explored, but only after "walking the walk" together. The process of mutual decision making, caring, and compassion over time is much more central to the care of the dying than the final act. The method used at the very end is relatively unimportant as long as it is consistent with the values of the persons involved. The personal commitment over time between patient, family, and health care provider is at the core. Jules, Judith, and Betty epitomized the ideal of what is possible.

Doctors, patients, and their families are engaged in negotiated deaths every day in every community in the United States. No one enjoys being involved in such processes. They are painful and unsettling even in the best of circumstances. Yet helping people die with their personhood intact is a fundamental responsibility of medical professionals. The final chapter in Jules's life illustrates the paradox of medicine's effectiveness in simultaneously prolonging life and creating new, more extreme forms of suffering. Medical technology is capable of tremendous good and terrible harm, depending on the patient's circumstances. Using it wisely is an awesome responsibility. We must learn to use it more judiciously and to stop it and be responsive when it no longer contributes to meaningful life. It is estimated that two-thirds of the six thousand deaths that occur each day in this country are negotiated and planned in some way. Our successes have created awesome new burdens for which we must share responsibility.

References

Medical Decisions That End Life Should Never Be Easy

Conwell, Y., and E. D. Caine. Rational suicide and the right to die: Reality and myth. *New England Journal of Medicine* 325 (1991): 1100–1103.

Gert, B., J. L. Bernat, and R. P. Mogielnicki. Distinguishing between patient's refusals and requests. *Hastings Center Report*, July–August 1994, 13–15.

Quill, T. E. Doctor, I want to die. Will you help me? *Journal of the American Medical Association* 270 (1993): 870–73.

———. When all else fails. *Pain Forum* 4 (1995): 189–91.

Quill, T. E., and C. K. Cassel. Nonabandonment: A central obligation for physicians. *Annals of Internal Medicine* 122 (1995): 368–74.

Quill, T. E., C. K. Cassel, and D. E. Meier. Care of the hopelessly ill: Proposed criteria for physician-assisted suicide. *New England Journal of Medicine* 327 (1992): 1380–84.

Rie, M. A. The limits of a wish. *Hastings Center Report*, July–August 1991, 24–27.

Potential Beauty of a Planned Process

Battin, M. P. Euthanasia: The way we do it, the way they do it. *Journal of Pain and Symptom Management* 6 (1991): 298–305.

———. *The Least Worst Death: Essays in Bioethics on the End of Life.* New York: Oxford University Press, 1994.

Eddy, D. M. A conversation with my mother. *Journal of the American Medical Association* 272 (1994): 179–81.

Jecker, N. S. Physician-assisted death in the Netherlands and the United States: Ethical and cultural aspects of health policy development. *Journal of the American Geriatrics Society* 42 (1994): 672–78.

Quill, T. E., and G. Kimsma. End-of-Life Care in the Netherlands and the United States: A Comparison of Values, Justifications, and Practices. Typescript.

Rollin, B. *Last Wish.* New York: Warner Books, 1985.

The Real Heroism in the Care of the Dying

Broadfield, L. Evaluation of palliative care: Current status and future directions. *Journal of Palliative Care* 4 (1988): 21–28.

Carlson, R. W., L. Devich, and R. R. Frank. Development of a comprehensive supportive care team for the hopelessly ill on a university hospital medical service. *Journal of the American Medical Association* 259 (1988): 378–83.

Cohen, S. R., and B. M. Mount. Quality of life in terminal illness: Defining and measuring subjective well-being in the dying. *Journal of Palliative Care* 8 (1992): 40–45.

Fulton, G. B., and E. K. Metress. *Perspectives on Death and Dying.* Boston: Jones & Bartlett, 1995.

Godkin, M. A., M. J. Krant, and N. J. Doster. The impact of hospice care on families. *International Journal of Psychiatry in Medicine* 13 (1983): 153–65.

Kane, R. L., L. Bernstein, J. Wales, and R. Rothenberg. Hospice effectiveness in controlling pain. *Journal of the American Medical Association* 253 (1985): 2683–86.

Mills, M., H. T. Davies, and W. A. Macrae. Care of dying patients in hospital. *British Medical Journal* 309 (1994): 583–86.

Nuland, S. B. *How We Die: Reflections on Life's Final Chapter.* New York: Knopf, 1994.

Rhymes, J. Hospice care in America. *Journal of the American Medical Association* 264 (1990): 369–72.

Volicer, L., Y. Rheaume, J. Brown, K. Fabiszewski, and R. Brady. Hospice approach to the treatment of patients with advanced dementia of the Alzheimer type. *Journal of the American Medical Association* 256 (1986): 2210–13.

Chapter 10

Partnership and Nonabandonment

PARTNERSHIP AND NONABANDONMENT are the core obligations of humane medical care for the dying. Debate in the United States about the role health care providers should play in their patients' deaths too often has been superficial and polarized. It is a debate between those who feel that patients have a "right to die" (as if dying were an option to be chosen) and those who believe that "easing death is too dangerous to vulnerable populations" (as if keeping suffering persons alive against their will protected them from abuse). One side does not hear the true anguish experienced by some dying patients, and the other side minimizes the real potential for life-ending clinical decisions to be adversely influenced by social factors. Despite the inherent complexity of life-and-death questions, patients and their families and doctors are struggling with them in the face of ethical, legal, and clinical uncertainty every day. The resolution of one complex ethical dilemma immediately raises two more. Since many patients end up in clinical situations that do not fit neatly into palliative care protocols, the physician's commitment not to abandon them in ethically gray circumstances is also pivotal. Therefore, the process of patient and physician working together in partnership over time may be more important than any specific question considered in isolation.

The conceptual models in this country of how death should be approached and what constitutes suffering are overly simplistic and woefully inadequate at the bedside. Death is often treated as an isolated event, and suffering is equated with physical pain, when, in truth, dying is a complex process that sometimes occurs in small increments over a very long period of time and suffering clearly includes a more comprehensive set of biological, psychological, social, existential, and spiritual dimensions. If our genuine interest is to better serve the needs of our dying patients, we must address a more complex set of questions, face some harder realities, and explore the messy middle ground between polarized positions. I therefore close with eleven challenges for patients, physicians, nurses, family members, ethicists, and policy makers as a starting point for a more meaningful discussion.[1]

1. *Physicians, nurses, and other health care providers who care for severely ill patients must become experts in comfort-oriented care.* Medical treatments geared to the relief of suffering and the maintenance of the quality of life are as central to the medical profession as those directed to the prolongation of life. Within the fields of hospice, palliative medicine, and pain management new techniques and effective strategies have been developed to relieve pain and other symptoms. Ignorance about modern methods of relieving symptoms or reluctance to administer opioid pain relievers are no longer acceptable excuses for withholding effective treatment from dying patients; it is a form of medical malpractice and should not be tolerated. No dying patients should want to end their life because they are not given access to currently available palliative treatments.

Similarly, a shift from aggressive, disease-oriented treatment to comfort-oriented care should be considered whenever suffering is extreme and the odds of treatment success are low. Even though Cynthia turned down comfort-oriented care when it was first offered early in her illness, choosing instead long-shot experimental therapy, it was an important and appropriate part of the discussion. Aggressive treatment was very unlikely to cure her cancer and would more likely aggravate rather than relieve her suffering. When her condition later worsened, Cynthia knew she had a meaningful alternative to the improbable fight for life she had initially chosen.

Many patients fear that they will be abandoned if they refuse med-

---

1. Recommended references for each challenge can be found at the end of the chapter.

ical care directed toward treating their underlying disease. Comfort care is the opposite extreme of abandonment. It involves intensive caring focused on the whole person, with special attention to promoting the quality of life, relief of suffering, and personal connection. It is a meaningful alternative to a death dominated by medical technology in which caring replaces curing as the dominant ethos. All physicians who work with severely ill patients must become skilled in its application, for it is the standard of care for the dying against which all other interventions should be measured.

Comfort care does more than address physical symptoms. Suffering is a complex amalgam of physical, psychological, social, spiritual, and existential elements, any of which may play a central role for a given patient. The nonphysical elements of suffering are unique to the individual and can be understood only by hearing the person's story. Sometimes the exploration of a patient's experience opens up avenues for intervention that no one could have anticipated. How could one possibly know that getting taxes done would be important to Jules, or that moving back into her own apartment would become essential to Mrs. Martinez, or that Native American chanting and drumming would be central to Robb's death? Sometimes simply listening to a story about which nothing can be done is the key intervention, lessening the aloneness of suffering.

In the United States, comfort care achieves its fullest expression in hospice programs, in which the resources of a multidisciplinary team including nurses, physicians, home health aides, social workers, clergy, and volunteers are available to address the various dimensions of a patient's suffering. To qualify, the dying patient must have a prognosis of six months or less and have a primary caregiver (usually a family member or friend) who is able to provide the bulk of the care and support at home. Initially hospice in the United States was exclusively home-based, but it has now been extended to nursing homes and small residential units for those without adequate home supports. Dedicated hospice workers help make dying more humane, and they have increased our knowledge about addressing the broad dimensions of human suffering.

The promise of hospice, that patients will not die alone or in pain, is welcomed and sufficient for most terminally ill patients. But as most hospice workers acknowledge, it is important not to overromanticize the process or to suggest that it will not be dominated by vexing challenges. Those who argue that all requests for physician-assisted death will be resolved by better pain relief do not do justice to the varied and complex problems with which the multidisciplinary hospice teams struggle on a daily basis. As Mr. Kline's story illustrates, not all pain can be relieved without unacceptable side effects (constipation, sedation, and delirium, to name a few), and treating terminal suffocation is taxing to everyone involved at the bedside even under the best of circumstances. The promise we make to our dying patients actually should have three parts: "You won't die alone, you won't die in pain, and we will struggle together to face whatever has to be faced." Most hospice workers make the latter commitment to confront the unknown together. If all physicians who care for severely ill patients would make this three-part commitment, much of the fear patients experience at the end of their lives would be lessened.

2. *We must learn how to talk openly with those who wish for death.* The wish for death frequently is expressed in intimate conversation with those who openly express their feelings about dying. In itself, it is certainly not a sign of psychopathology. Most often it is a natural part of the dying process, as with Mrs. Martinez, who was readying herself to join her beloved husband, or Mr. Williams, who found himself more deteriorated than he could have imagined after initially benefiting from his implantable defibrillator. Sometimes the wish for death is a cry for help, a sign of the desire to stop aggressive therapy and make the transition to comfort care or perhaps the sign of an emerging family crisis. At other times it is indicative of clinical depression darkly distorting one's perceptions, perhaps amenable to psychotherapy or antidepressant medication.

The meaning of a wish to die can be discovered only through open conversation. These discussions are often avoided in part because of our own discomfort as caregivers. Being in immediate proximity with such suffering is painful and frightening, particularly if one feels obligated to resolve it. Yet one can relieve a considerable amount of suffering simply by having the courage to listen and accept. Recall how alone Mr. Williams and Bill felt until someone finally was willing to take their lament seriously. No matter how one feels about assisting a patient to die, it is critical to explore the wish to die when it emerges in the patient's conversation. Even if all one can do is listen, at least the dying person is no longer alone with his or her thoughts and feelings. Most often the dialogue opens up avenues that are helpful but never reach the frightening ground of assisting death.

3. *Patients need an open-ended commitment from their physicians to help them find acceptable solutions to the vexing problems of dying.* Late at night, in the dark, when they are completely alone, many dying patients imagine their worst-case scenario. Jane would think about her experience with Bill, and Robb would see the many friends he had witnessed in the final stages of AIDS dementia. Knowing that there is the potential for escape if one should have the misfortune to experience his or her worst nightmare can be very important. Many dying patients spend their final time living in fear that they will be trapped in an unacceptable state with no possibility of release. Their psychic and spiritual energy is depleted by apprehension about future suffering rather than focused on the more important tasks of resolving unfinished business, putting their lives in perspective, and saying good-bye to those they love. When modern palliative techniques are used, most patients' fears will not come to fruition. Nonetheless, without the knowledge that one will be allowed an escape under the harshest of circumstances, one's final days can be dominated by dread rather than hope.

The knowledge that one's physician will respond to the extremes of suffering can be very reassuring and even liberating. In Cynthia's case, it initially helped her find the courage to try experimental therapy and then gave her peace of mind for the month she spent on hospice before her death. For Jules, Betty's commitment that "when the time comes for you to die, and you are completely sure, I will be there for you and help you as best I can" freed him to keep living and try life-prolonging treatments that he never thought he would be able to tolerate. Later, when he was disheartened about how diminished his life had become, picking a date when his ordeal would be ended and knowing that his doctor would be there for him gave him the energy to prepare himself and his family for his death.

The absence of this commitment is part of our core problem in the care of the dying. Many dying patients do not feel that they can count on their doctors to be responsive when and if they begin to live out their worst nightmare, especially if it falls outside of rigidly prescribed legal and ethical boundaries. As the stories in this book illustrate, the complex realities of dying patients rarely remain entirely within these confines. This fear is probably a potent force behind the drive to legalize physician-assisted dying in the United States. Perhaps doctors would be more committed and flexible in their partnerships with patients if the legal prohibitions were taken out of the equation. Somehow, we must create an atmosphere in which it is not only legally safe but also professionally and morally mandatory to make this commitment.

4. *Dying patients should be given as much choice and control as possible according to the limitations of their disease.* Patients have little control over where their illnesses are ultimately taking them, but they should be given the widest possible range of options about how to get there. The principles of autonomy and self-determination underlie this fundamental precept. Most hospice programs pride themselves on keeping their patients in the driver's seat, providing as many choices as possible rather than imposing rigidly prescribed regimens. Most patients make good decisions when they are given this freedom and power. They are thereby better able to put their own unique stamp on the final chapter of their life. It is arrogant and presumptuous to think that health care providers, hospice workers, and ethicists know how to write it for them.

Many of these same dedicated professionals believe that dying patients should not be given the possibility of choosing death, no matter how terrible their circumstances. A line is drawn in the sand, and the motivations of the dying patient and the receptive physicians begin to be questioned if they contemplate crossing it. It is argued that such patients must be depressed or have unresolved, pathological needs to control the uncontrollable. Doctors who are willing to assist must be doing so because of their own psychic weakness or professional inexperience. Yet six of the nine patients whose stories are included here reached the point where, having explored and understood all the alternatives, they wanted to die. In most cases, their wish could be accommodated using standard palliative care strategies, though sometimes the edges had to be tested. Except for Mr. Williams, all had the reassuring commitment that if their suffering became overwhelming, a mutually acceptable answer would be found.

Yet some solutions presented in these stories were clearly better than others. Both Jules and Jane died planned deaths after long struggles with progressively worsening diseases that left them severely depleted. Both were surrounded by friends who loved them dearly. Both feared suffocation and needed to be given a large dose of sedatives in order not to struggle. Unfortunately, because Jane did not have a life-sustaining treatment to discontinue, her act had to be carried out in secret. When things went wrong and it appeared that she might not have taken enough medicine to ensure her death, there was no doctor there to help her over the threshold. Her friends fulfilled their commitment to Jane, but their actions caused them considerable pain, undermining the love and caring that was otherwise demonstrated. I feel as if I abandoned Jane and her friends and that our years of partnership were severely compromised. Jane was allowed to maintain her integrity while completing her life story, but her friends and I remain haunted that she had to die with a plastic bag over her head. There is no place for such stark images in a humane system of caring for the dying.

5. *Physicians must be fully educated about currently accepted options for easing death.* Approximately two-thirds of deaths in the United States each day involve the doctor's participation, at least indirectly. Opioid pain-relievers and/or sedatives are often used at the end of a long illness

to relieve terminal suffering in doses that indirectly contribute to a wished-for death (Cynthia, Mrs. Martinez, Robb, Mr. Kline, and Jules). Patients also have the right not to start life-sustaining treatment (Mrs. Johnson, Robb) or to discontinue it when it no longer meets their goals (Cynthia, Mr. Kline, Jules). These decisions are basic matters of informed consent and include instances when patients are motivated by a clearly articulated wish to die. There is simply no reason why patients like Mr. Williams should have to beg or even attempt suicide in order to have their requests taken seriously. Patients who have chosen to forgo or stop life-sustaining therapy often require aggressive symptom-relieving measures during the dying process, so the two methodologies outlined above often need to be combined in practice. These interventions that indirectly help patients to die have wide medical, ethical, and legal acceptance. Doctors and other health care providers must become proficient at offering them and then carrying them out.

Terminal sedation with barbiturates or benzodiazepines has recently been added as an optional relief measure for patients suffering in dimensions other than pain. As the case of Mr. Kline illustrates, heavy sedation can be used when patients develop delirium or other kinds of anguish that cannot be relieved with opioids. The intent is to relieve intolerable suffering, and the patient is then "allowed to die" of a combination of the underlying disease, the sedation, and dehydration. Similarly, patients may stop eating and drinking under the rubric of the "right to refuse treatment" and then be "allowed to die" of dehydration and the underlying disease. The physician's role is considered ethically passive, ensuring informed consent and then easing any suffering that emerges as the process unfolds.

If terminal sedation and voluntary dehydration are to be the options of last resort, offered to patients who want to die despite comprehensive palliative care, then we should educate physicians about their acceptability. Such means of escape explicitly acknowledge what patients and their families already know: that some dying patients reach a point where their misery is so irreversible and grim that they prefer dying to continued suffering. Terminal sedation and voluntary dehydration provide a means of dying to all suffering patients, not just those in severe physical pain or those dependent on life-sustaining therapy. Whenever any life-ending treatments are considered, a second opinion should be obtained to ensure that all palliative care alternatives have been explored. Since these interventions result in the patient's death, we will need to be very clear about their moral and legal acceptability before physicians feel confident about using them. For patients and families who have witnessed physicians turning their backs on patients whose suffering did not fit into neat palliative care protocols, these would be reassuring additions.

6. *We must be sure that the current ethical distinctions between "active" and "passive" assisted dying and between physician-assisted suicide and euthanasia are clinically meaningful and morally worth preserving.* All medical interventions that will result in the patient's death, whether direct or indirect, intended or unintended, should be the interventions of last resort. In my view, the specific method used is much less important than the process of caring, excellent palliative care, and joint decision making that precede it. If a potentially life-ending intervention is needed, it should be consistent with the values of the particular patient and physician, especially if it involves their joint participation. In most circumstances, the patient's closest family should also be involved, since they will have to make sense of the process in the future. Concepts like the "double effect" may be pivotal in determining some individuals' decisions, whereas to others these distinctions seem self-deceptive and meaningless. The primary intention of any and all potentially life-ending physician intervention must always be to relieve the patient's suffering. Unfortunately, some patients find the final relief only in their death.

Mr. Kline was treated with terminal sedation as a last resort to fulfill our promise that he would not die an agonizing death. He was put under the equivalent of general anesthesia and then "allowed to die" from dehydration. The difference between terminal sedation and euthanasia (when a lethal overdose is given at the terminally ill patient's request) is paper thin, requiring a highly intellectualized analysis and presentation of the physician's intentions. In both circumstances, the patient inevitably dies as a result of the treatment. With terminal sedation, the wished-for death must be *foreseen* but not *intended* if it is to remain under the protective umbrella of the "double effect." The potential for self-deception in such justifications is substantial.

All the risks cited for sanctioning physician-assisted suicide and euthanasia apply to terminal sedation, since it too is a life-ending treatment (intended or not). Any of these three interventions could clearly be used for humane purposes, and just as clearly abused. In order to distinguish between them, we must always look at both the practical and the theoretical implications. Terminal sedation has an implicit safeguard built in because it requires involvement of the health care team, but it has the disadvantage of requiring that the patient dehydrate to death over several days in an iatrogenic coma. For some patients and families, this final period is a time for quiet reflection and closure, and for others it may only add a final humiliation to their already overwhelming losses. We must learn to ask hard questions about all potentially life-ending treatments and not assume that some categories are inherently safe and others are immoral by definition.

In the United States, a sharp distinction is being made between physician-assisted suicide (in which the physician provides a lethal medicine that the patient can take on his or her own) and voluntary euthanasia (in which the physician provides a lethal injection at the patient's explicit request). If we are eventually to legalize some form of physician-assisted death, the patient's ability to carry out the final act independently is felt to be an important safeguard to ensure voluntariness. Although I don't believe these acts are morally distinct, the practical differences are important. If we as a society choose to allow physician-assisted suicide but not voluntary euthanasia, we must require that the physician be available and empower the physician to respond to potential problems. An oral overdose of barbiturates is lethal within five hours in about 80 percent of cases, provided it is given in an adequate dose.[2] Some of the remaining 20 percent of patients may need some additional assistance to die peacefully. It is not fair to put family and friends in the position of having to use a plastic bag or to force a patient to reawaken to a life already devoid of meaning in an even more compromised condition. If we choose to allow physician-assisted suicide but not voluntary euthanasia, we must think through all the practicalities. The partnership between doctor and patient must continue throughout any life-ending process if we are to fulfill our commitment not to abandon.

7. *Safeguards must be defined and implemented for any and all treatments that result in a patient's death.* Although there are important distinctions to be made between the methods illustrated in these chapters, many of them facilitate a wished-for death. All decisions having such profound consequences must be made entirely in the patient's best interests, as free as possible of adverse external influences. For this reason, all such interventions, whether they be sedating doses of pain-relieving opioids, discontinuance of life-sustaining treatment, terminal sedation, voluntary dehydration, or more explicit forms of physician-assisted death (physician-assisted suicide or voluntary euthanasia), should incorporate safeguards. These safeguards would include the following: *(a)* the patient must be fully informed about his condition, prognosis, and treatment choices, including more conventional comfort-care options; *(b)* the patient's thinking must be clear and rational, and a psy-

---

2. The only good published data on this topic come from the Netherlands, where physician-assisted death remains illegal but is openly tolerated provided one acts within carefully defined safeguards. The Dutch have more than twenty years of experience with the open practice of euthanasia and physician-assisted suicide, including close cooperation between physicians and pharmacists. Data about the efficacy of an oral barbiturate overdose are from P. V. Admiraal, Toepassing van euthanatica, *Netherlands Tydschrift voor Geneeskunde* 139 (1995): 265–68. A recent report of the experience from Compassion in Dying, a Washington State–based group that counsels patients who request physician-assisted suicide and then accompanies those who meet their criteria, suggests an efficacy rate closer to 100 percent (T. A. Preston and R. Mero, Observations concerning terminally ill patients who choose suicide, *Journal of Pharmaceutical Care in Pain and Symptom Control* 4 [1996]: 183–92).

chiatrist should be consulted if there is potential distortion by depression or other mental disorder; *(c)* the patient's suffering must be unbearable, and all reasonable palliative care alternatives must be at least considered and, preferably, tried; *(d)* the patient must have a terminal disease; *(e)* an independent second opinion should be obtained from a person knowledgeable about palliative care to verify that each of the above criteria has been met.

Restricting the possibility of a physician-assisted death to terminally ill patients involves a tradeoff between the safety of limiting the practice to those who are close to death with or without medical intervention and withholding it from suffering patients with incurable but not imminently terminal illnesses, in which cases the risk of error is greater. The practice should initially be restricted to this group because of current inequities of access to health care, the changing medical market place, and our lack of experience with an open process. If, in the future, physician-assisted death is to be extended to incurably ill but not imminently terminal patients, safeguards for these incurably ill patients will need to be even more stringent, including longer waiting periods and mandatory assessments by psychiatrists, specialists, and those who have expertise in palliative care. In the interim we must work creatively with our incurably ill, suffering patients to ensure that they receive the best of palliative care, including adequate management of pain and symptoms, good social supports, and freedom from unwanted medical intervention.

Discussion about increased options for dying patients to actively choose death if their suffering becomes intolerable should be conducted only in the context of excellent comfort-oriented care. Allowing physician-assisted death to be an alternative to good medical care would be immoral and unthinkable. Any intervention that results in a patient's death should be offered only as a last resort, after all reasonable comfort-oriented options have been exhausted. Any proposal considering legitimization of physician-assisted death should require access to comprehensive palliative care as a precondition. The physician providing a second opinion must have extensive experience in caring for the dying. Allowing patients to choose death makes sense only as the final expression of our caring and obligation not to abandon, not as an alternative to the best medical care available.

8. *The main public policy question is whether patients would be better served by safeguards controlling a more explicit, open process than they are by the current unstated policy requiring secrecy and ambiguity whenever death is eased.* Throughout the United States each day doctors, patients, and their families are involved in death-related decision making, not because they want to be, but because they have to be. Our successes in keeping patients alive longer have created new dilemmas that would have been inconceivable in the past. Sometimes, as with Mr. Kline's implantable defibrillator, the standard principles of medical ethics can resolve the question (i.e., patients have the right to discontinue any treatments that do not serve their goals). But at other times our successes have increased the probability of patients' literally falling apart before they die—disintegrating as human beings from the relentless progression of their disease and its treatment.

All the patients whose stories are presented here used modern medicine to live longer. Most eventually made an active decision to stop treatment and then took advantage of excellent hospice care. However, they also used supplementary methods to end their lives when their suffering became extreme. It is impossible to consciously hasten death and stay within the confines of the "double effect." In this religiously based doctrine, intentionally shortening life is immoral by definition, no matter how bleak and irreversible the patient's circumstances. Yet for many suffering persons who have outlived their natural life span death is not unwelcome. After using modern medicine to help patients live longer, more meaningful lives, we have a responsibility to help them find death when continued living becomes excruciating in spite of our best efforts to comfort them.

The current requirement that easing death always be unintentional, indirect, or covert is dangerous for patients and erodes the integrity of the professions of medicine and law. Most medical professionals learn to couch their actions under the inherent ambiguity of the "double effect." If one chooses to respond explicitly to a patient's request for aid-in-dying, one must act in secret without the benefit of consultation or open decision making, hedging one's intentions or lying outright about what has transpired. Even when medical examiners and prosecutors discover the physician-assisted suicide of a terminally ill patient, they usually do not pursue it as long as there is no evidence of foul play and the media is not involved. Most understand that there is no need to put a family already grieving over the loss of a loved one through an additional legal ordeal.

The potential risks of a more open process must also be carefully considered. The United States is a technology-driven society obsessed with cost containment. The Social Darwinism evident in Washington might be all too willing to embrace physician-assisted death as a money-saving alternative to universal access to good medical care. Vulnerable patients might be subtly or explicitly coerced to choose death over expensive medical treatment or custodial care. Patients might feel a "duty to die" without spending the family inheritance or expanding the national debt. Our society might be only too willing to choose a quick, inexpensive, technical solution to the often messy process of dying. Our health care system may be too anonymous, episodic, and variable to ensure the delicate, intimate decision making described in this book. These risks are real and substantive.

The questions for policy makers, health care providers, and citizens are whether the risks of changing public policy can be adequately contained with carefully crafted safeguards and whether dying patients are really autonomous enough to make good decisions for themselves even when saddled with complex illness. I believe a more open process is better for patients and doctors than the current policy, where the safest approach from a legal perspective is to walk away from difficult end-of-life problems, leaving the patient and family to either continue suffering or act on their own. Doctors who refuse to abandon their patients must now act in secret or else learn how to hide their actions within the confines of the "double effect." A more explicit, forthright, open public policy that ensured informed consent, access to comfort-oriented care, and an independent second opinion would surely be better than this. If we choose not to change public policy, we must still decide how to respond to our dying patients whose suffering becomes intolerable without giving them false reassurance, turning our backs, or requiring deception and secrecy. There is no risk-free way to proceed, but our patients clearly are telling us that our current approaches are inadequate.

9. *Managed care has the potential to disrupt the long-term patient-doctor relationship so central to end-of-life decision making.* Health care in the United States is undergoing radical reform, driven more by the need to control costs than by principles of improving quality and access. Even though the United States spends more per capita on health care than any other Western nation, the uninsured population now numbers forty million and continues to grow. There is little talk in Washington about how to erase this national shame. Instead, "for-profit" market forces are being allowed to use money saved by reducing some of the system's excesses to reward investors and increase corporate profits. Without a clearly defined commitment to universal access to good quality care, reform may reduce the medical profession to a commodity made up of interchangeable pieces that can be bought and sold.

Yet, this transformation also provides the opportunity to both improve the quality of care and contain costs for the dying. Overuse of medical technology at the end of life continues to be widely documented, sometimes even when it means ignoring the wishes of the patient and the family for a less aggressive approach.[3] Managed care systems could reinforce hospice care as the standard of care for the dying and discourage the use of futile, death-denying technological interventions. Hospice care allows potential for both cost saving and quality improvement in the care of the dying.

Furthermore, patients in managed care systems could be encouraged to complete living wills and health care proxies (see the Appendix

3. See The SUPPORT Principle Investigators. A controlled trial to improve care for seriously ill hospitalized patients: The study to understand prognoses and preferences for outcomes and risks of treatment (SUPPORT), *JAMA* 274 (1995): 1591–98.

for instructions and sample forms). Then, in the event that a patient became mentally incapacitated, his or her values and expectations regarding death would be known in advance. The system could then help ensure that such directives would be honored, not allowing doctors to unilaterally override them in a monolithic fight for life. By recommitting to providing the dying with better choices and more assurance that their values will drive treatment, we would have the opportunity to both improve quality and save money. If our commitment becomes dominated by cutting costs, then the risk of explicitly or covertly coercing patients to die prematurely will be increased. Assisted dying by direct or indirect measures must never become an alternative to the best palliative care available.

Managed care also has the potential to strengthen or weaken the doctor-patient relationship. On the potentially positive side, most patients will have the vast majority of their care flow through a primary care physician who can help them decide how to access the complex medical systems. Instead of being cared for by multiple specialists, each attending to one organ system but often not considering the overall person, the primary care physician will be responsible for working with the patient to oversee the overall care plan. There will also be incentives for primary care doctors to help control overall costs by practicing according to agreed-upon quality standards. If such systems encourage intimate, long-term relationships between primary care doctors and patients and more appropriate utilization of effective treatments, they might improve the overall quality of health care. However, if cost-saving incentives to these physicians are too strong and access to specialists is too restricted, the potential for conflict of interest will be substantial. Furthermore, if patients are forced to choose between competing health plans with different providers each year, as has happened in many health care "markets," this could undermine the entire fabric of personal medical care. In order for medical treatment to be best used in a personalized way, considerable trust and shared experience have to be developed over time.

Many of the stories in this book were based upon long-term doctor-patient relationships (Robb, Mrs. Martinez, Mrs. Johnson, John, Mr. Kline, Jane). The shared experience that predated their final illness provided a context of trust and intimacy that allowed a wider range of discussion and higher-quality decision making than might otherwise have been possible. Wide cultural and ethnic barriers between myself and Mrs. Martinez and Mrs. Johnson were successfully bridged before challenging end-of-life decisions had to be made. Such continuity of care needs to be preserved in our efforts at health care reform. However, given our mobile society and the rapidly changing health care systems, such continuity may not always be possible. Intimate, person-centered care is still feasible even if doctor and patient first come to know each other in the midst of a severe illness, provided doctors have proper training in both communication skills and palliative care. I first met Cynthia after she had been diagnosed with her ultimately terminal illness, and our relationship spanned only a few months. Betty became Jules's primary care doctor when his ALS was already far advanced, yet they were able to face the hardest of decisions together. I saw Mr. Williams only once, yet I was able to help him along his path by listening and learning about his dilemma with the implantable defibrillator with an open mind and then by using my knowledge about palliative care and medical ethics. No matter what system of health care eventually is put in place, we will still have a professional obligation as individual physicians to address the circumstances faced by the patients and families who come under our care. Health care will always be a very human endeavor. If our society sacrifices in-depth human engagement between doctors and patients in an effort to save money, we will lose something very precious.

10. *A bad death should be considered a medical emergency.* Dying patients need health care providers who will face the future with them no matter what happens. Most of the time, the careful application of comfort care principles and techniques helps patients to achieve a death that is tolerable if not always ideal. Infrequently, patients reach a point at which they seek death because they feel humiliated and sense that they are disintegrating as persons with no other escape. This state of

being is fundamentally disturbing to patients, families, and caregivers. Although it is not always within our power to resolve such an experience, it should be considered a medical emergency that requires an immediate, creative response. In the intensive care unit, when a person's life is at stake we show no restraint in acting on the patient's behalf. We must demonstrate that same immediacy and lack of restraint in the midst of bad death, when the patient's personhood is at stake. In such cases, we must use all our personal and medical resources to find a solution that is acceptable to the patient. It is the ultimate expression of our commitment not to abandon the dying.

The rights of dying patients to an assisted death are not unlimited, nor are the concomitant obligations of their physicians. Patients have a right to *request*, but not to *demand*, a physician-assisted death. Their doctors are obliged to understand exactly what is being requested, to explore why it is being requested at a particular point in time, and then to search for palliative care possibilities. If there are no acceptable alternatives, doctors should have the freedom to assist the patient to die as a last resort if it is consistent with their value structure. If a physician cannot respond directly because of moral or religious principles, the physician is still obligated to work with his or her patient to find a mutually acceptable solution. Simply saying no without making a diligent, creative effort to find alternatives is not adequate. Such desperate cries for help cannot go unheeded by a medical profession that takes seriously its duty to relieve unbearable human suffering.

II. *Nonabandonment is fundamental to the long-term doctor-patient partnership.* Nonabandonment reinforces a longitudinal commitment that is an essential aspect of being a physician and is too often inadequately captured in traditional ethical analyses. Patients seek physicians who will make the commitment both to care about and know them as persons and to be their guides and partners in sickness and health until their death. In this context, patients and physicians can learn to judiciously use medicine's power and expand the concept of healing to include working with persons with severe chronic illnesses and disabilities as well as persons who are dying. The commitment not to abandon supplements the caring relationship because it requires that the physician and patient work together over time, even when the path is unclear. Moral challenges must be met and engaged in with the patient, not shied away from by recourse to falsely bright lines or unbending rules. There is a world of difference between facing an uncertain future alone and having a caring partner who will be present no matter what happens.

Such partnerships between physicians and patients are at the core of the medical profession. They must be explicitly represented in the discourse of medical ethics, creating an important tension between the worlds of abstract principles and real patients. Physicians and other health care providers who find that their work with patients has lost its excitement and meaning would do well to consider engaging in these types of relationships. Health planners, legislators, risk managers, medical educators, and ethicists should carefully examine whether their contribution to health care tends to reinforce or obstruct such commitments. Clinical medicine is ultimately a humbling and exhilarating profession, filled with joy, sorrow, and an overabundance of uncertainty that comes with establishing a genuine long-term connection with patients. To practice medicine with a commitment to caring and to be there no matter what the future holds is to experience the richness of the human condition over and over again and to know one has made a difference. If the obligation of nonabandonment is centrally incorporated into medical ethics, medicine may become more humanized and more responsive to the problems faced every day by patients, their families, and their physicians.

It is fitting to close with a patient's perspective, as eloquently articulated by Cynthia in an interview conducted about one week after her ultimately fatal illness was first diagnosed:

> The kind of doctor-patient relationship that is healing and helpful for me is one where the doctor becomes a partner, and where what we do together is seen in a much larger way than simply, "I am going to cure you of this disease or not." . . . It is that kind of larger heal-

ing relationship that has to do with me as a person going through something rather than me as a disease that has a certain course. This has really helped me find the space to make some decisions and begin to move with this. . . . that sense of my doctors being people—human people in a human relationship with me. And that you are fallible. While on the one hand, I don't want you to be fallible, on the other, I know that's the case. If it is an acknowledged part of the relationship, that opens up all kinds of vistas, all sorts of possibilities of hope for me. Because if you can't do everything for me that I would like you to do or that you would like to do, that doesn't mean that we are at the end of the road. If I know that, and we work together, and it gets to the point that we are at the end of this road, and you are still there to help me explore other roads, then it makes the whole process a lot more—well, in some ways wonderful, and certainly a lot more tolerable.

References

Expertise in Comfort Care

American Board of Internal Medicine. *Caring for the Dying—Identification and Promotion of Physician Competency: Personal Narratives.* Philadelphia, 1996.

Enck, R. E. *The Medical Care of Terminally Ill Patients.* Baltimore: Johns Hopkins University Press, 1994.

Foley, K. M. The treatment of cancer pain. *New England Journal of Medicine* 313 (1989): 84–95.

Garfield, C. A. *Psychosocial Care of the Dying Patient.* New York: McGraw-Hill, 1978.

Patt, R. B., ed. *Cancer Pain.* Philadelphia: J. B. Lippincott, 1992.

Quill, T. E. *Death and Dignity: Making Choices and Taking Charge.* New York: W. W. Norton, 1993.

Saunders, C., and N. Sykes, eds. *The Management of Terminal Malignant Disease.* 3d ed. London: Edward Arnold, 1993.

Wallston, K. A., C. Burger, R. A. Smith, and R. J. Baugher. Comparing the quality of death for hospice and non-hospice cancer patients. *Medical Care* 26 (1988): 177–82.

Talking Openly about the Wish to Die

Ackerman, F. The significance of a wish. *Hastings Center Report*, July–August 1991, 27–29.

Baron, R. J. An introduction to medical phenomenology: I can't hear you while I'm listening. *Annals of Internal Medicine* 103 (1985): 606–11.

Block, S. D., and J. A. Billings. Patient requests to hasten death: Evaluation and management in terminal care. *Archives of Internal Medicine* 154 (1994): 2039–47.

Eddy, D. M. A conversation with my mother. *Journal of the American Medical Association* 272 (1994): 179–81.

Quill, T. E. Doctor, I want to die. Will you help me? *Journal of the American Medical Association* 270 (1993): 870–73.

Rie, M. A. The limits of a wish. *Hastings Center Report*, July–August 1991, 24–27.

Zinn, W. The empathic physician. *Archives of Internal Medicine* 153 (1993): 306–12.

Open-Ended Commitment between Doctors and Patients

Jecker, N. S. Giving death a hand: When the dying and the doctor stand in a special relationship. *Journal of the American Geriatrics Society* 39 (1991): 831–35.

Novack, D. H. Therapeutic aspects of the clinical encounter. *Journal of General Internal Medicine* 2 (1987): 346–55.

Peabody, F. W. The care of the patient. *New England Journal of Medicine* 88 (1927): 877–82.

Quill, T. E. Partnerships in patient care: A contractual approach. *Annals of Internal Medicine* 98 (1983): 228–34.

Quill, T. E., and C. K. Cassel. Nonabandonment: A central obligation for physicians. *Annals of Internal Medicine* 122 (1995): 368–74.

Respecting and Promoting Individual Choice

Blackhall, L. J., S. T. Murphy, G. Frank, V. Michel, and S. Azen. Ethnicity and attitudes toward patient autonomy. *Journal of the American Medical Association* 274 (1995): 820–25.

Brody, D. S. The patient's role in clinical decision making. *Annals of Internal Medicine* 93 (1980): 718–22.

Callahan, D. When self-determination runs amok. *Hastings Center Report*, March–April 1992, 52–55.

Gostin, L. O. Informed consent, cultural sensitivity, and respect for persons. *Journal of the American Medical Association* 274 (1995): 844–45.

Kassirer, J. P. Adding insult to injury: Usurping patients' prerogatives. *New England Journal of Medicine* 308 (1983): 898–901.

Lomas, H. D. Paternalism: Medical or otherwise. *Social Science and Medicine* 15F (1981): 103–6.

Quill, T. E. Partnerships in patient care: A contractual approach. *Annals of Internal Medicine* 98 (1983): 228–34.

Varki, A. Of pride, prejudice, and discrimination: Why generalizations can be unfair to the individual. *Annals of Internal Medicine* 116 (1992): 762–64.

Currently Accepted Options for Easy Death

General References

American College of Physicians. American College of Physicians Ethics Manual, 3d ed. *Annals of Internal Medicine* 117 (1992): 947–60.

American Medical Association's Council on Ethical and Judicial Affairs. Decisions near the end of life. *Journal of the American Medical Association* 276 (1992): 2229–33.

Council on Scientific Affairs, American Medical Association. Good care of the dying patient. *Journal of the American Medical Association* 275 (1996): 474–78.

Gostin, L. O., and F. R. Weir. Life and death choices after Cruzan: Case law and standards of professional conduct. *Milbank Quarterly* 69 (1991): 143–73.

Hastings Center. *Guidelines on the Termination of Life-Sustaining Treatment and the Care of the Dying.* New York, 1987.

President's Commission for the Study of Ethical Problems in Medicine and Biomedical and Behavioral Research. *Deciding to Forego Life-Sustaining Treatment: A Report on the Ethical, Medical, and Legal Issues in Treatment Decisions.* Washington, D.C.: U.S. Government Printing Office, 1983.

Wanzer, S. H., S. J. Adelstein, R. E. Cranford, D. D. Federman, E. D. Hook, C. G. Moertel, P. Safar, A. Stone, H. B. Tausig, and J. van Eys. The physician's responsibility toward hopelessly ill patients. *New England Journal of Medicine* 310 (1984): 955–59.

Wanzer, S. H., D. D. Federman, S. J. Adelstein, C. K. Cassel, E. H. Cassem, R. E. Cranford, E. W. Hook, B. Lo, C. G. Moertel, and P. Safar. The physician's responsibility toward hopelessly ill patients: A second look. *New England Journal of Medicine* 320 (1989): 844–49.

Withholding and Withdrawing Treatment

Edwards, M. J., and S. W. Tolle. Disconnecting a ventilator at the request of a patient who knows he will then die: The doctor's anguish. *Annals of Internal Medicine* 117 (1992): 254–56.

Glantz, L. Withholding and withdrawing treatment: The role of the criminal law. *Law, Medicine and Health Care* 15 (1988): 231–41.

Meisel, A. Legal myths about terminating life support. *Archives of Internal Medicine* 151 (1991): 1497–502.

Miller, D. K., R. M. Coe, and T. M. Hyers. Achieving consensus on withdrawing or withholding care for critically ill patients. *Journal of General Internal Medicine* 7 (1992): 475–80.

Terminal Sedation

Cherny, N. I., and R. K. Portenoy. Sedation in the management of refractory symptoms: Guidelines for evaluation and treatment. *Journal of Palliat Care* 10 (1994): 31–38.

Quill, T. E., and R. V. Brody. "You promised me I wouldn't die like this": A bad death as a medical emergency. *Archives of Internal Medicine* 155 (1995): 1250–54.

Truog, R. D., C. B. Berde, C. Mitchell, and H. E. Grier. Barbiturates in the care of the terminally ill. *New England Journal of Medicine* 327 (1991): 1678–81.

Terminal Dehydration

Andrews, M., E. R. Bell, S. A. Smith, J. F. Tischler, and J. M. Veglia. Dehydration in terminally ill patients: Is it appropriate palliative care? *Postgraduate Medicine* 93 (1993): 201–3.

Bernat, J. L., B. Gert, and R. P. Mogielnicki. Patient refusal of hydration and nutrition: An alternative to physician-assisted suicide or voluntary active euthanasia. *Archives of Internal Medicine* 153 (1993): 2723–28.

Eddy, D. M. A conversation with my mother. *Journal of the American Medical Association* 179 (1994): 179–81.

McCann, R. M., W. J. Hall, and A. Groth-Juncker. Comfort care for terminally ill patients: The appropriate use of nutrition and hydration. *Journal of the American Medical Association* 272 (1994): 1263–66.

Pearlman, R. A. Forgoing medical nutrition and hydration: An area for fine-tuning clinical skills. *Journal of General Internal Medicine* 8 (1993): 225–27.

Printz, L. A. Terminal dehydration, a compassionate treatment. *Archives of Internal Medicine* 152 (1992): 697–700.

Sullivan, R. J., Jr. Accepting death without artificial nutrition or hydration. *Journal of General Internal Medicine* 8 (1993): 220–24.

Limitations of Current End-of-Life Distinctions

Brock, D. W. Voluntary active euthanasia. *Hastings Center Report*, March–April 1992, 10–22.

Brody, H. Causing, intending, and assisting death. *Journal of Clinical Ethics* 4 (1993): 112–17.

Devettere, R. J. The imprecise language of euthanasia and causing death. *Journal of Clinical Ethics* 1 (1990): 268–77.

Kamm, F. M. The doctrine of double effect: Reflections on theoretical and practical issues. *Journal of Medical Philosophy* 16 (1991): 571–85.

Marquis, D. B. Four versions of the double effect. *Journal of Medical Philosophy* 19 (1991): 515–44.

Quill, T. E. The ambiguity of clinical intentions. *New England Journal of Medicine* 329 (1993): 1039–40.

Rachels, J. Active and passive euthanasia. *New England Journal of Medicine* 292 (1975): 78–80.

Safeguards for all Life-Ending Treatments

Alpers, A., and B. Lo. Physician-assisted suicide in Oregon: A bold experiment. *Journal of the American Medical Association* 274 (1995): 483–87.

Baron, C. H., C. Bergstresser, D. W. Brock, G. F. Cole, N. S. Dorfman, J. A. Johnson, L. E. Schnipper, J. Vorenberg, and S. W. Wanzer. Statute: A Model state act to authorize and regulate physician-assisted suicide. *Harvard Journal on Legislation* 32 (1996): 1–34.

Brody, H. Assisted death—a compassionate response to a medical failure. *New England Journal of Medicine* 327 (1992): 1384–88.

Compassion in Dying v. State of Washington No. 94–35534, 1996 WL 94848 (9th Cir., 6 March 1996).

Miller, F. G., T. E. Quill, H. Brody, J. C. Fletcher, L. O. Gostin, and D. E. Meier. Regulating physician-assisted death. *New England Journal of Medicine* 331 (1994): 119–23.

Quill, T. E., D. E. Meier, F. G. Miller, B. Lo, and D. Brock. Physician-assisted death: A comparison of terminal sedation, physician-assisted suicide, and voluntary active euthanasia. Typescript.

Public Policy Debate

Brody, H. Assisted death—a compassionate response to a medical failure. *New England Journal of Medicine* 327 (1992): 1384–88.

Cassel, C. K., and D. E. Meier. Morals and moralism in the debate over euthanasia and assisted suicide. *New England Journal of Medicine* 323 (1990): 750–52.

Fins, J. J., and M. D. Bacchetta. Framing the physician-assisted suicide and voluntary active euthanasia debate: The role of deontology, consequentialism, and clinical pragmatism. *Journal of the American Geriatrics Society* 43 (1995): 563–68.

Foley, K. M. Pain, physician-assisted suicide, and euthanasia. *Pain Forum* 4 (1995): 163–78.

Kamisar, Y. Against assisted suicide—even a very limited form. *University of Detroit Mercy Law Review* 72 (1995): 735–69.

Lee, M. A., and S. W. Tolle. Oregon's assisted suicide vote: The silver lining. *Annals of Internal Medicine* 124 (1996): 267–69.

Miller, F. G., and J. C. Fletcher. The case for legalized euthanasia. *Perspectives in Biology and Medicine* 36 (1993): 159–76.

Miller, F. G., T. E. Quill, H. Brody, J. C. Fletcher, L. O. Gostin, and D. E. Meier. Regulating physician-assisted death. *New England Journal of Medicine* 331 (1994): 119–23.

Quill, T. E., C. K. Cassel, and D. E. Meier. Care of the hopelessly ill: Potential criteria for physician-assisted suicide. *New England Journal of Medicine* 327 (1992): 1380–84.

Teno, J., and J. Lynn. Voluntary active euthanasia: The individual case and public policy. *Journal of the American Geriatrics Society* 39 (1991): 827–30.

Managed Care at the End of Life

Cassel, C. K. The patient-physician covenant: An affirmation of Asklepios. *Annals of Internal Medicine* 124 (1996): 604–6.

Emanuel, E. J., and A. S. Brett. Managed competition and the patient-physician relationship. *New England Journal of Medicine* 329 (1993): 879–82.

Morrison, R. S., and D. E. Meier. Managed care at the end of life. *Trends in Health Care, Law and Ethics* 10 (1995): 91–96.

Rodwin, M. A. Conflicts in managed care. *New England Journal of Medicine* 332 (1995): 604–7.

Sulmasy, D. P. Managed care and managed death. *Archives of Internal Medicine* 155 (1995): 133–36.

A Bad Death Is a Medical Emergency

Quill, T. E., and R. V. Brody. "You promised me I wouldn't die like this": A bad death as a medical emergency. *Archives of Internal Medicine* 155 (1995): 1250–54.

Nonabandonment

American Board of Internal Medicine. *Caring for the Dying—Identification and Promotion of Clinical Competency: Educational Resource Document.* Philadelphia, 1996.

Cassell, E. J. *The Nature of Suffering and the Goals of Medicine.* New York: Oxford University Press, 1991.

Council on Scientific Affairs, American Medical Association. Good care of the dying patient. *Journal of the American Medical Association* 275 (1996): 474–78.

Peabody, F. W. The care of the patient. *New England Journal of Medicine* 88 (1927): 877–82.

Quill, T. E. *Death and Dignity: Making Choices and Taking Charge.* New York: W. W. Norton, 1993.

Quill T. E., and C. K. Cassel. Nonabandonment: A central obligation for physicians. *Annals of Internal Medicine* 122 (1995): 368–74.

Wanzer, S. H., S. J. Adelstein, R. E. Cranford, D. D. Federman, E. D. Hook, C. G. Moertel, P. Safar, A. Stone, H. B. Tausig, and J. van Eys. The physician's responsibility toward hopelessly ill patients. *New England Journal of Medicine* 310 (1984): 955–59.

Wanzer, S. H., D. D. Federman, S. J. Adelstein, C. K. Cassel, E. H. Cassem, R. E. Cranford, E. W. Hook, B. Lo, C. G. Moertel, and P. Safar. The physician's responsibility toward hopelessly ill patients: A second look. *New England Journal of Medicine* 320 (1989): 844–49.

Appendix

Advance Directives
Health Care Proxy and Living Will

W HAT FOLLOWS WAS obtained from Choice In Dying, Inc., 200 Varick Street, New York, N.Y. 10014. Advance-directive requirements may vary slightly from state to state but are generally transferable. State-specific forms can be obtained from Choice In Dying at 1-800-989-WILL[*]

This packet contains two legal documents that protect your right to refuse medical treatment you do not want, or to request treatment you do want, in the event you lose the ability to make decisions yourself:

1. The New York Health Care Proxy lets you name someone to make decisions about your medical care, including decisions about life support, if you can no longer speak for yourself. The Health Care Proxy is especially useful because it appoints someone to speak for you any time you are unable to make your own medical decisions, not only at the end of life.

2. The New York Living Will lets you state your wishes about medical care in the event that you develop an irreversible condition that prevents you from making your own medical decisions. The Living Will becomes effective if you become terminally ill, permanently uncon-

[*] Reprinted by permission of Choice In Dying, 200 Varick Street, New York, NY 10014, 212/366-5540.

scious or minimally conscious due to brain damage and will never regain the ability to make decisions.

Choice In Dying recommends that you complete both of these documents, to best ensure that you receive the kind of medical care you want when you can no longer speak for yourself.

Note: These documents will be legally binding only if the person completing them is a competent adult (at least 18 years old).

The New York Health Care Proxy

Whom Should I Appoint As My "Proxy"?

A "proxy" (or "agent") is the person you appoint to make decisions about your medical care if you become unable to make those decisions yourself. The person you name as your proxy should clearly understand your wishes, and be willing to accept the responsibility of making medical decisions for you. Your agent can be a family member or a close friend whom you trust to make these serious decisions.

The person you appoint as your agent cannot be:

1. an operator, administrator or employee of a health care facility in which you are a resident or patient, or to which you have applied for admission, at the time you sign your proxy, unless that person is a relative by blood, marriage or adoption;

2. a physician, if that person also acts as your attending physician; or

3. anyone who is already an agent for ten or more people, unless that person is related to you by blood, marriage or adoption.

You can also appoint a second person as your alternate proxy. The alternate will step in if the first person you name as proxy is unable, unwilling, or unavailable to act for you.

How Do I Make My New York Health Care Proxy Legal?

The law requires that you sign and date your Health Care Proxy in the presence of two adult witnesses. The witnesses must sign a statement in your Health Care Proxy to confirm that you signed the document willingly and free from duress. The person you name as your agent or alternate agent cannot act as a witness.

In addition, if you are a resident in a facility operated or licensed by the office of mental health or the office of mental retardation and developmental disabilities, there are special witnessing requirements. Contact Choice In Dying for more information.

Choice In Dying also recommends that you avoid having your relatives, or other beneficiaries of your estate, act as witnesses.

Note: You do not need to notarize your New York Health Care Proxy.

Should I Add Personal Instructions to My New York Health Care Proxy?

Choice In Dying advises you to add only one statement to this document: "My agent knows my wishes concerning artificial nutrition and hydration." This statement is necessary because of a specific provision in the law that allows your agent to authorize the withholding or withdrawal of tube feeding only if he or she knows that you would wish to refuse it.

We recommend that you not add any other statements because you might unintentionally restrict your proxy's power to act in your best interests. One of the strongest reasons for naming a proxy is to have someone who can respond flexibly as your medical situation changes, and can deal with situations that you did not foresee.

Instead, we urge you to talk with your agent about your future medical care, and to describe what you consider to be an acceptable "quality of life." If you want to record your wishes about specific treatments or conditions, you should use the New York Living Will.

What If I Change My Mind?

You may revoke your Health Care Proxy by notifying your proxy or a health care provider orally or in writing of your revocation, or through any other act that clearly shows your intent to revoke the document. A physician who is informed of your revocation must record the revocation in your medical record and notify the proxy and any medical staff responsible for your care.

The New York Living Will

How Do I Make My New York Living Will Legal?

The New York Living Will is authorized by law created by New York courts, not by legislation. For this reason, there are no specific requirements guiding its use. Choice In Dying recommends that you follow the witnessing procedures established in the Health Care Proxy Act and sign your Living Will in the presence of two adult witnesses, who should not be beneficiaries of your estate.

Note: You do not need to notarize your New York Living Will.

Can I Add Personal Instructions to My Living Will?

Yes. You can add personal instructions in the part of the document called "Other directions." For example, if there are any specific forms of treatment that you wish to refuse that are not already listed on the document, you may list them here. Also, you can add instructions, such as "I do not want to be placed in a nursing home," or "I want to die at home."

If you have also appointed a proxy, it is a good idea to write a statement such as, "Any questions about how to interpret or when to apply my Living Will are to be decided by my proxy."

Note: It is important to learn about the kinds of life-sustaining treatment you might receive. Consult your doctor or order the Choice In Dying pamphlet, "Medical Treatments and Your Living Will."

What If I Change My Mind?

If you decide to cancel your Living Will, follow the same procedures outlined for revoking your Health Care Proxy.

What to Do after You Have Completed Your Documents

Your New York Health Care Proxy and New York Living Will are important legal documents. Keep the original signed documents in a secure, but accessible place. Do not put the original forms in a safe deposit box or any other security box that would keep others from having access to them.

2. Give photocopies (xerox copies) of the signed originals to your proxy and alternate proxy, to your doctor(s), family, close friends, clergy and anyone else who might become involved in your health care. If you enter a nursing home or hospital, have photocopies of your documents placed in your medical records.

3. Be sure to talk to your proxy (and alternate), your doctor(s), clergy, and family and friends about your wishes concerning medical treatment. Discuss your wishes with them often, particularly if your medical condition changes.

4. If you want to make changes to your documents after they have been signed and witnessed, you must complete new documents.

5. Remember, you can always revoke one or both of your New York documents.

6. Please be aware that your New York documents will *not* be effective in the event of a sudden emergency. Ambulance personnel are required to provide CPR (cardiopulmonary resuscitation) unless they are provided with a separate "Non-Hospital Do Not Resuscitate (DNR) Order." If this concerns you, ask your doctor or local hospital for more information about a Non-Hospital DNR Order, or contact Choice In Dying. If you would like to receive an actual Non-Hospital DNR *form,* call the New York State Department of Health at (518) 474-7354.

New York Health Care Proxy

(1) I, _____, hereby appoint:

(name)

_____

(name, home address and telephone number of proxy)

_____

as my health care agent to make any and all health care decisions for me, except to the extent that I state otherwise.

This Health Care Proxy shall take effect in the event I become unable to make my own health care decisions.

(2) Optional instruction: I direct my proxy to make health care decisions in accord with my wishes and limitations as stated below, or as he or she otherwise knows.

(Unless your agent knows your wishes about artificial nutrition and hydration [feeding tubes], your agent will not be allowed to make decisions about artificial nutrition and hydration.)

(3) Name of substitute or fill-in proxy if the person I appoint above is unable, unwilling or unavailable to act as my health care agent:

_____

(name, home address and telephone number of alternate proxy)

_____

(4) Unless I revoke it, this proxy shall remain in effect indefinitely, or until the date or condition I have stated below. This proxy shall expire (specific date or conditions, if desired): _____

_____

_____

(5) Signature_____ Date_____

Address_____

Statement by Witnesses (must be 18 or older)

I declare that the person who signed this document is personally known to me and appears to be of sound mind and acting of his or her own free will. He or she signed (or asked another to sign for him or her) this document in my presence. I am not the person appointed as proxy by this document.

Witness 1_____

Address_____

Witness 2_____

Address_____

New York Living Will

This Living Will has been prepared to conform to the law in the State of New York, as set forth in the case In re Westchester County Medical Center, 72 N.Y.2d 517 (1988). *In that case the Court established the need for "clear and convincing" evidence of a patient's wishes and stated that the "ideal situation is one in which the patient's wishes were expressed in some form of writing, perhaps a 'living will.'" (Cross out any statements with which you disagree.)*

I, _____, being of sound mind, make this statement as a directive to be followed if I become permanently unable to participate in decisions regarding my medical care. These instructions reflect my firm and settled commitment to decline medical treatment under the circumstances indicated below:

I direct my attending physician to withhold or withdraw treatment that merely prolongs my dying, if I should be in an **incurable or irreversible mental or physical condition with no reasonable expectation of recovery.**

These instructions apply if I am (a) **in a terminal condition;** (b) **permanently unconscious;** or (c) **if I am minimally conscious but have irreversible brain damage and will never regain the ability to make decisions and express my wishes.**

I direct that my treatment be limited to measures to keep me comfortable and to relieve pain, including any pain that might occur by withholding or withdrawing treatment.

While I understand that I am not legally required to be specific about future treatments **if I am in the condition(s) described above I feel especially strongly about the following forms of treatment:**

I do not want cardiac resuscitation.
I do not want mechanical respiration.
I do not want artificial nutrition and hydration.
I do not want antibiotics.

However, **I do want** maximum pain relief, even if it may hasten my death.

Other directions:

These directions express my legal right to refuse treatment, under the law of New York. I intend my instructions to be carried out, unless I have rescinded them in a new writing or by clearly indicating that I have changed my mind.

Signature_____ Date_____

Address_____

I declare that the person who signed this document is personally known to me and appears to be of sound mind and acting of his or her own free will. He or she signed (or asked another to sign for him or her) this document in my presence.

Witness 1_____

Address_____

Witness 2_____

Address_____

TIMOTHY E. QUILL is a professor of medicine and psychiatry at the University of Rochester School of Medicine and Dentistry in Rochester, New York. He heads the university's Program for Biopsychosocial Studies and was a hospice medical director for eight years. He is currently the associate chief of medicine at the Genesee Hospital, where he has been in primary care practice for sixteen years. His research and teaching interests include the doctor-patient relationship, partnership, communication, somatization, medical ethics, palliative care, and end-of-life decision making.

He is best known for his 1991 *New England Journal of Medicine* narrative about "Diane," a woman dying of leukemia to whom he provided a prescription of barbiturates so that she could have more choice in determining how much suffering was enough. Dr. Quill is a staunch advocate of hospice care as the standard of care for all dying patients, but he also believes that we must be more responsive when and if hospice care fails to adequately relieve a person's suffering. With this in mind, he has published clinical safeguards for more openly responding to those terminally ill suffering patients who want physician-assisted suicide as a last resort, and he is the lead plaintiff in a lawsuit *(Quill v. Vacco)*, recently heard in the United States Court for the Second Circuit, in which the laws prohibiting physician-assisted suicide were found to be unconstitutional. This ruling, and a similar case from the Ninth Circuit, on the West Coast, are currently being appealed to the United States Supreme Court.

Library of Congress Cataloging-in-Publication Data

Quill, Timothy E.
A midwife through the dying process : stories of healing and
hard choices at the end of life / Timothy E. Quill.
p.   cm.
ISBN 0-8018-5516-0 (alk. paper)
1. Assisted suicide. 2. Right to die. 3. Terminal care.
I. Title.
R726.Q55   1996
179'.7—dc20   96-26475
CIP

Printed in the United States
3585